MW01225712

STIRRUPS

STIRRUPS

What Every OB/GYN Should Tell You, But Doesn't

Stefanie,
Good to see you again at
Karen & Randy's.
Best wishes on your upcoming
wedding & future,

Eban H. Rock, MD

Eban H. Rock, MD
aka Harold

ORANGE *frazer* PRESS
Wilmington, Ohio

ISBN 978-1939710017
Copyright©2013

No part of this publication may be reproduced in any material form (including
photocopying or storing in any medium by electronic means and whether or not
transiently or incidentally to some other use of this publication) without the written
permission of the copyright holder except in accordance with the provisions of the
Copyright, Designs and Patents Act 1988.

Published for the author by:
Orange Frazer Press
P.O. Box 214
Wilmington, OH 45177
Telephone: 800.852.9332 for price and shipping information.
Website: www.orangefrazer.com
www.orangefrazercustombooks.com

Book and cover design: Brittany Lament and Orange Frazer Press

Library of Congress Control Number 2013935248

To my former patients who trusted me enough to confide in me and tell me their innermost feelings, desires, and satisfactions, and allowed me to care for them, their loved ones, and their friends.

TABLE OF CONTENTS

X

STIRRUPS

PREFACE

This book is written for women. After thirty-four years of caring for, talking to, questioning, and especially listening to women and believing what they told me, I learned much about their perceptions and misperceptions about their bodies, their physiology, psychology, and their sexuality. This is my effort to provide clear and understandable information that I hope will relieve women of worry and guilt and help them realize they are normal. In addition, I have included information about pregnancy, labor and delivery, anesthesia, sexuality, and various medical conditions to enable them to make informed choices. Technical details, treatment modalities, and personal philosophy for the practice of ob/gyn are included for residents and practitioners.

In many cases I have used descriptions of actual patient encounters—with the names changed—to illustrate the issues. These are true stories about real patients and I write this under a nom de plume to further insulate these patients from identity. I extend my apologies to any former patients that might feel offended or embarrassed when reading their case history, albeit under another name. To them I say: Please realize how much your story will help other women with the same condition or problem and forgive me for causing you discomfort. I plead with anyone to whom these identities as well as my identity may be apparent not to divulge them, so that your sisters or friends may remain anonymous.

ACKNOWLEDGMENTS

Writing under a nom de plume has a huge downside. Most of the people who gave me great assistance must go unidentified. There were many, starting with my high school guidance counselor, who made me realize that I could become a doctor. My family, especially my grandparents and aunts, who housed and fed me through my college years, were around long enough to see me become established and successful. My mother and siblings gave me all the support they could, and I can never repay them. My wife was incredibly supportive and spent so many nights and weekends without me to help raise the family. What an incredible job she did, as evidenced by the success of our grown children and their success in raising our grandchildren.

As is very evident, I owe my former patients an everlasting debt of gratitude for teaching me things I could have learned in no other way. Their trust and willingness to confide in me is the reason for this book. One former patient, in particular, read parts of the early manuscript, was encouraging, and gave me guidance on how to go about getting published.

The attentiveness of my residents and the stimulation they gave me to remain up to date in the specialty was invaluable. It is extremely gratifying to have seen so many become successful, assume positions of leadership, and be highly respected by their peers.

The people at Orange Frazer Press, Marcy Hawley and staff, were unstinting in their encouragement and expertise in helping a writing—and computer—challenged physician create something readable. Editor John Baskin was incredibly helpful and patient as he helped me construct the manuscript.

INTRODUCTION

I began the private practice of obstetrics/gynecology as
the third member of an established group practice. My first
day in the office coincided with the first day of my senior
partner's six-week vacation. For the next six weeks, all of the
post-partum (six-week checkup) patients I saw were patients
he had delivered, verified by his trademark mediolateral
episiotomy scar that extended from the bottom of the vaginal
opening into the right buttock. My training had emphasized
the median episiotomy, straight back in the midline, which
healed more quickly, had less blood loss, and was far less
painful. Those advantages hold even if the incision must be
extended to incise the anal canal (episioproctotomy), as long
as it is properly repaired.

After six weeks of this, and running late during a very busy
day, I entered the exam room and greeted a patient already
on the table. I introduced myself, sat down on the stool, and
observed a thin, well-healed midline scar.

"Oh," I said, looking up at her between her legs, "I
delivered you!"

She sat bolt upright with her feet still in the stirrups,
pointed at my face, and exclaimed, "Now I know what they say
about you obs is true—that you only know your patients by
their bottoms."

Whoops! What could I say and how did I get there?

As one of eight children growing up in a government project, our family was poor but not much worse off than the other residents of the village. This was post-Depression middle America, and the entire middle class was poor. An exception was the village doctor who lived next door. Even by the age of seven, I was aware of how admired and respected he was. It never entered my mind that I could be a doctor.

During my third year of high school, a new guidance counselor appeared on the scene and did vocational testing for my class of forty-five students. By then I was working evenings and weekends at the village pharmacy. I had started there as a soda jerk, been promoted to the drugstore side, then advanced to apprentice pharmacist. I met with Miss Gundle to discuss the results of the test.

"Eban," she asked, "what do you want to be?"

I told her that I thought maybe I could be a pharmacist.

"Eban," she said, "you can be anything you want to be. Have you ever thought about being a doctor?"

Wow! That totally shocked me. I expressed doubt, but she convinced me that I could do it. I only had to figure out how.

I knew that I was on my own and there was no possibility of financial support. By then my father, who suffered with what is now called bipolar disease, had become an unreliable provider. He later committed suicide. I worked many jobs from then until I was well into my residency. Most summers I had three jobs, for example: full-time day laborer for the local park board; 6 to 11 p.m. weeknights at the local creamy whip store; and weekends at the delicatessen. During my college years I worked as a drugstore clerk, supermarket cashier, and at the university on an Air Force project. During my residency, I was locum tenens for some family practitioners, covering for their vacations. In my last year of residency I was on call, in the hospital, every other night, working thirty-six hours on, twelve hours off. I moonlighted on my nights off, covering anesthesia.

During my senior year in high school, I applied to a university in a nearby city and over four years completed an excellent premed course. Despite all the jobs, I graduated near the top of my class. I did get major support during college, living with and being fed by my grandparents and two spinster aunts who lived a mile from campus. Accommodations were a little sparse and warm. My basement bedroom was in a former coal bin and my desk was next to the gas-fired furnace.

I applied to three medical schools and was accepted by all. I matriculated at the first-tier school in my home city and lucked out on a great job. Starting the summer before entry, I got "on the job training" at a hospital a block from the medical school, taking x-rays and electrocardiograms. I did this every fourth night (all night as needed) and every fourth weekend. It paid room and board and $25 a month. I also worked at another hospital as an ob extern every sixth night, assisting at deliveries and surgeries. After my second year, I took a two-week training course in nursing and worked summers as the charge nurse at the medical school hospital.

I married at the end of that first year. We lived in government subsidized public housing. I took an x-ray job at the hospital where I was working as an ob extern. I was paid

$125 a month, without the room and board. I scheduled the work so that every twelfth night I worked both jobs on the same night, which I did for the next three years. I was paid out of two different cost centers and never got caught, nor did I ever have a situation where patients in serious need had to wait for my services. My thanks go out to the nurses in the emergency department and labor and delivery who for short periods made excuses for me.

We were the first occupants of a small two-bedroom apartment in a new section of the public housing project. It was nice but the neighbors left more than a little to be desired. One close neighbor often called in her five children with, "All you little bastards, get your asses in here." We subsequently found out that having five different fathers, they were all bastards.

The rent for the first year, based on my income, was $27 a month. During the next year of medical school, with clinical rotations, I had to spend nights on call at the hospital. I couldn't work as much so, and as my income fell, our rent dropped to $19 a month.

It wasn't as hard as it sounds. You tackle problems and difficulties one at a time and then forget them. We were happily married and young and strong. There was, however, one rough spot that I will never forget. By the time I entered internship we had two children. In the last month of medical school, with final exams and the state board exam to take, I had to quit my jobs. I had taken student loans during medical school and was $15,000 in debt. In today's dollars, that is probably more than $50,000.

The internship, at the hospital where I had been working, paid monthly. By the middle of July we ran out of money and had no food in the house. I told my wife not to worry—I would get an advance on my pay for the two weeks that I had worked. Surprise, surprise! They wouldn't give it to me. I appealed, telling the paymaster my story and reminding him that I had been a faithful hospital employee for the last three years. Still no! A short time later I was in the office of the CEO, a doctor who was also the head of the department of anesthesiology.

He listened to my plea and said, "I'm sorry, Dr. Rock, I just cannot set a precedent like that." I was crying as I went up to the medical education office, worried about going home without groceries and what I was going to tell my wife. The director of medical education asked what was wrong. I explained and he asked if a loan of $100 would hold me until payday, then wrote me a check.

A month later, I inadvertently got a bit of payback. I was the intern on a large (fifty-six bed) medical unit. Toward mid-afternoon the unit charge nurse said to me, "Dr. Rock, you are taking care of our sickest patients. Do you think they will do all right tonight with just an LPN in charge."

"What are you talking about?" I asked.

"With the nursing shortage," she said, "there is no RN available. The RN from the adjacent unit will come over to give the meds, but otherwise there will be no nurse."

"That's ridiculous," I said, "and just asking for trouble." I said that I had had training as a nurse after my second year in medical school and had worked the previous summer as the charge nurse on a terminal tumor and urology ward at the medical school hospital. I told her that if they would pay me special duty nurse rates, I would work that night.

A short time later, I was called to the office of the hospital head nurse. She questioned me about my nurse's training and experience, thought for a minute or so, and finally said, "I don't think that will do, Dr. Rock, but thank you for offering."

At that point, I became angry. I was really worried about two of my sickest patients. "Do you mean to tell me that you think those patients will be better off with an LPN in charge rather than a doctor with nursing training and experience?" I said. "I wonder what our metropolitan newspaper would think about that."

Twenty minutes later, I was back in the CEO's office with the head nurse. Dr. CEO asked about my experience, then asked the head nurse to question me.

"Dr. Rock," she asked, "if you were to report for duty, how would you conduct yourself? What would you do?"

Nurses have a checklist they go through at the beginning of each shift, and I knew it cold. I rattled it off. Holding her hands apart, palms up, she gave Dr. CEO an imploring look. I was dismissed to wait in the outer office. A short time later, they hired me.

The night was busy, but serving as both doctor and nurse was very efficient. I didn't have to call anyone else the entire night. Thirty-six dollars was the going rate for a special duty shift. That wasn't why I did it, but it helped. They called me many times over the next few months, asking me to work this unit or that. I declined them all.

I was concentrating on my internship.

STIRRUPS

STIRRUPS

CHAPTER ONE

Office Routines and Pregnant Patients: How to Counsel the Ladies

My specialty is primarily an office practice specialty. There is surgery and delivering babies, of course, but the bulk of my time is spent seeing patients for problems they are having, for contraception or routine annual checkups. Yearly Pap smears, we now know, are not necessary for most women but serve the laudable purpose of bringing patients in once a year when a complete physical can be done. Many ob/gyn specialists only do a breast and pelvic exam, but it's my strong feeing that the checkup should be more complete. We are often the only doctor that women of this age see on a regular basis. It only takes a few additional minutes to check the eyes, ears, nose and throat, to palpate the thyroid, listen to the heart and lungs, palpate the abdomen, feel for enlarged lymph nodes, and inquire of the patient about any problems. For all new and yearly checkup patients, this was my routine physical.

Women who are planning to start a pregnancy, as well as women who may think that they are not but are having unprotected sex, should be careful about several things. To them I say that you need to be sure that you have a healthy diet, especially with regard to leafy green vegetables, citrus fruit, and probably animal products, which will provide folic acid. It is well established that folate deficiency at the time of conception results in a higher incidence of neural tube defects—spina bifida and hydrocephalus—in babies. I routinely put all my patients on prenatal vitamins containing folic acid for this reason. These women should also review all their medications for pregnancy contraindications. Recreational drugs, excessive alcohol, and smoking are too risky for the fetus.

Women need to know about the spontaneous miscarriage rate. It runs about 15 percent (one in seven) from the time a woman is a week or so late for a period and realizes that she is pregnant. Sensitive pregnancy tests may diagnose pregnancy a week after conception, well before the next expected menstrual period, and at that time the miscarriage risk is closer to 20 percent (one in five). I warned these patients not to tell everybody in the world they are pregnant that early, because it's a bad job to have to tell them that you lost it.

I told all my patients contemplating pregnancy that early miscarriages (before twelve weeks from the last period, assuming a twenty-eight day cycle) are programmed to happen at the moment of conception, with only very rare exceptions. I explained that sometimes the egg is a little old, or the sperm a little defective, or maybe they just don't come together right.

Many times a fetus doesn't even form, and it is just placental tissue that produces pregnancy hormones.

This is critical for women to know because the bleeding that announces the start of the miscarriage always begins right after she did something, such as lifting something heavy, exercising, or—heaven forbid—having sex. The latter occurs often because intercourse, especially if orgasm occurs, causes the uterus to contract, and if there is any loose blood in there it is going to come out. Not knowing this causes many women to suffer with intense guilt that can carry over into the next pregnancy, causing undue concern and needless precautions.

Women need to know that a bad pregnancy can't be kept and a good one can't be gotten rid of—short of a direct attack such as scraping or sucking it out or poisoning it. To my more worldly patients I would say, "You can screw them in but you can't screw them out." Those tiny fetuses are tenacious and healthy ones are impervious to a woman's ordinary activities, and that includes vigorous sex. If they were that easy to get rid of there wouldn't be abortion clinics.

I saw many wonderful patients in my office, and I learned so much from them. Starting private practice in a group practice also gave me the opportunity to learn from my partners. One thing that I learned early in my career was how to deal with overweight pregnant patients. This I discovered after hearing patients describe their feelings after seeing one of my partners on a previous visit. That partner was very stern with patients with excessive weight gain, threatening that dire medical problems would result if they didn't control the weight. This routine upset patients because they were already concerned about their additional weight gain during pregnancy and frustrated trying to deal with it. One told me that she became so upset that she stopped at the dairy store on the way home and had a double hot fudge sundae.

Doctors, in my view, should never frighten patients to try and get them to comply with instructions. Patients usually already know about the consequences. If I was asked about the risks, I generally minimized the danger because I knew their minds would exaggerate it. It's much more effective to let the patient know how it would please you, the doctor, if they changed to a healthier practice. I became convinced that it was totally counterproductive to even mention weight to a pregnant women. Once I decided on this course, though, I had to persuade my office nurses to join in. My head nurse would raise an eyebrow to her hairline when she had to slide the weight on the scale arm clear to the end. That had to stop.

Bringing up the subject proved to be unnecessary because every one of these ladies would, on their fourth or fifth month visit, ask me something like, "Doctor, is my weight going to be a problem?" My response was that it is an overrated problem; we once thought excessive weight gain caused an increase in toxemia of pregnancy, with high blood pressure and other problems. We now know that this increase occurs primarily in very obese women.

"Obese patients can be a little harder to care for," I would say. "Getting an accurate blood pressure, picking up the fetal heartbeat, and feeling the baby's position can be harder to do." If

I was feeling mischievous that day I might say, "It can be a little harder to start an IV and get a good epidural in." That might be perceived as a little threat, but I so enjoyed watching their eyes open wide, and I knew what they were thinking: Sheesh, harder to get a good epidural; I better stop eating so much!

Having this opening, I could continue my counseling. "Now that you have reached this point in pregnancy you probably don't have to eat every fifteen minutes to prevent nausea, so it might be a good idea to try to stop eating anything between meals, as well as reducing the portion size. You will be much happier with yourself after delivery and motivated to get back to your previous figure." This approach gave better results than the more directive method.

Admittedly, it was much harder to care for obese patients than those of more normal weight. Everything was harder to do. Sewing up an episiotomy on a really obese patient is one of the hardest jobs I did. It made for really tired fingers. It was easy to make the cut with the baby's head distending the mother's bottom, but when the baby is out and the extra fat is pushing everything together, you have to pry it apart to sew it together. Yes, there are retractors for that, but they are cumbersome and slow you down.

I must confess that when I was having a fat day in the office, I would sometimes total up the weight of patients and go whining to my receptionist, "Mary Jane, what did I do to you? Why are you treating me like this? Do you know how many tons of patients you've scheduled for me today?" Her response was always, "Get out of my office."

One of my most pleasant patients, with her first pregnancy, was in for her fourth visit. She was twenty-one years old, just over five feet tall, and weighed over two hundred pounds. She asked me the question, and I gave her my standard response. Then she said, "Dr. Rock, you are so nice. I have a friend who is fat like me and her doctor is terrible to her. He told her that if he were her husband he would divorce her. I said, 'You should go to my doctor. He loves fat women!'"

My head nurse nearly knocked over her chair getting out of the exam room.

CHAPTER TWO

Anesthesia and Natural Childbirth: First-class Deliveries

While covering for another obstetrician, the department chairman who was out of town, his patient Lydia went into labor. I first met her and her husband at 2 a.m. as she was admitted to the labor room. It was her second pregnancy; she was in good labor and feeling a lot of pain. She loved her epidural, and we all enjoyed the recording of Rachmaninoff's Piano Concerto No. 2 that her husband tuned up. Her doctor returned the next day and provided her postpartum care.

Time passed, and three years later, running a little behind, I opened the patient's chart as I entered my exam room. She was a beautiful brunette whom I didn't recognize; the chart was blank. A cold chart, I called it—something my nurse was going to hear about.

The patient saw my confusion and said, "You don't remember me, do you, Doctor?"

I stammered and lied. "Well, you look familiar," I said.

"Dr. Rock," she said, "after I spend an entire night with a man, I don't expect him to forget me."

It was Lydia, back for her third pregnancy. She had several more babies and, in addition, sent me many wonderful patients, and her memorable delivery—verbal and otherwise— allowed me to segue into the new procedures developed during my medical training in the 1960s, some of which I was able to popularize in my home city. Two of these procedures involved obstetric anesthesia—the use of spinals and epidurals, which were almost unavailable from anesthesiologists because of the bad hours and paltry insurance remuneration. Most patients were then relegated to a general anesthetic, which was given by nurse anesthetists. Spinals were given only by doctors, usually the obstetrician or a resident physician. Epidurals came on the scene later.

In my internship hospital, obstetric anesthesia was so neglected, in fact, that you could seldom get an anesthesiologist— even during business hours—to ride the elevator eight floors up from surgery to the labor floor to give a spinal. The department chief (the hospital CEO) was especially difficult. Nurse anesthetists, assigned to labor and delivery, gave only general anesthetics in those days and, as they were in short supply, their coverage was spotty. As a result, after a well-taught, one-month rotation with these same anesthesiologists, I was giving spinal and general anesthetics for the delivery of private patients.

It was something I really enjoyed. It was tremendously gratifying to relieve a patient's pain, especially for women undergoing such a momentous and usually happy event. I seriously considered choosing anesthesiology as my specialty, but I already loved delivering the babies too much.

One of the techniques I learned was how to give spinal anesthesia with a very thin, 26-gauge needle that virtually eliminated post spinal headaches. These headaches are caused by leakage of spinal fluid from the puncture hole in the dural sac into the surrounding tissue. The brain floats in spinal fluid and if the fluid is reduced, it sags and pulls on the cranial nerves when the patient assumes an upright position, causing a very characteristic headache.

When, as a brand new first-year resident in a different hospital, I introduced this technique to its busy maternity service, it increased the use of this very safe and effective anesthetic and allowed many women to witness the birth. Prior to that time, spinals were routinely given with a stiffer, thicker 22-gauge needle, which was much easier to use but had the disadvantage of a 15 percent incidence of post-spinal headaches in postpartum patients. The problem was compounded by the infrequent use of IVs during labor, resulting in dehydrated patients. In addition, one of the postpartum floors was not air conditioned. At the start of my residency on July 1, there were always three or four patients spending extra days in the hospital, lying flat in bed to relieve their headaches.

The nurses called on me often to give spinals to patients. They were mostly private patients, and I enjoyed monitoring their vital signs as their obstetrician delivered them. I was a rather cheeky first-year resident, and if I nailed the spinal on the first attempt with the smaller needle, which I did about 95 percent of the time, I made it a point to give the patient—with her obstetrician listening—some postpartum instructions.

"When you get to the postpartum floor the nurses are going to tell you that you must lie flat," I said, "not even raise your head for twelve hours or you will get a spinal headache. You tell the nurse that Dr. Rock gave you the spinal and that you can get up anytime you want to. Do have help the first time out of bed because you might be a little unsteady."

I always enjoyed the look on the attending obstetrician's face, but none of the patients got a headache. It's virtually impossible for a postpartum patient not to raise her head, for instance, when she uses the bedpan, and if the patient got a headache the doctor deflected blame to the patient by saying that she must have raised her head. A lot of blame-deflecting goes on in medicine, and I hate it. I always felt that the doctor should accept responsibility for his or her actions and, in addition, should warn the patient of potential side effects. For instance, I told patients that their midline episiotomy would hurt in the rectal area for twelve to twenty-four hours. Postpartum nurses usually inspect episiotomies and often attribute any pain to hemorrhoids rather than the doctor's repair.

"You don't have hemorrhoids," I told my patients. "It's my stitches."

In the second year of my residency, an attending obstetrician admitted a doctor's wife in labor and gave her a continuous epidural. I had never heard of this. I assisted him and marveled at the results—a painless wide-awake labor and delivery, familiar these days to most women. As far as I know, he never gave another epidural, but I couldn't stop giving them.

My first, under that obstetrician's supervision to a clinic patient, worked well and gave me an instant reputation with the nurses. During the last year of my training, I was on call in the hospital every other night (thirty-six hours on, twelve hours off). On my nights off—if I wasn't already there moonlighting covering anesthesia—I occasionally got called in from home to give an epidural to a nurse, doctor, or other VIP for the labor and delivery. Of course, I gave many while on duty.

Years later, in private practice with my two partners, epidurals were the order of the day (and night). To do this, we agreed to go to the hospital when we sent the patient because if you waited until the nurse called to confirm labor, you would often arrive too late to give one. This requirement, combined with the anesthesia department's neglect, kept us the only game in town for several years, until increasing demand by other obstetricians and hospital administrators forced anesthesia departments to provide the service.

Our practice grew rapidly. Beauty parlors were our unpaid advertisers. In those days, a new mother would get a hairdo as soon as possible after delivery, and we would get a bunch of calls for new patient appointments. Of course, giving epidurals required that we spend an enormous amount of time at the hospital because the procedure required constant monitoring, re-dosing, and attention. Patients got the benefit of having the doctor there for the entire labor, and because they were wide awake and comfortable, we began to allow the husband to remain in attendance for the labor and delivery. It's hard to believe that back then the father had to wait in the "fathers' waiting room" the entire time, usually not seeing his wife from admission until she was rolled out with the baby.

Then there is natural childbirth. I learned many things from my patients—things not found in books and not taught in medical school. One early discovery was that some patients have no pain at all during labor or delivery. I learned this first from a patient I saw in the intern's clinic. She was perhaps seventeen, unmarried, and living with an elderly spinster aunt in a cold water, walk-up flat. Her father, a minister in a small town seventy miles from the city, had thrown her out when her pregnancy was discovered. She missed most of the childbirth classes because she had to work. She had nothing going for her but guilt and anxiety. I spent a lot of time giving her support and encouragement during her prenatal visits.

On my call night, I spotted her being wheeled into the labor admitting room. She greeted me and said that she was glad that I was on call.

"Are you in labor?" I asked.

"No," she said, "but I am having contractions and my water broke so I thought I should come in."

About two minutes later the nurse hurried out of the admitting room and announced, with a look of disbelief, "She is ready for delivery."

We took her to the delivery room and, in my ignorance, I gave her a spinal and she had an easy delivery. The anesthetic, as I learned from subsequent patients during my residency, was unnecessary. Because she was so pain free in labor, she would not have had pain with the delivery, either.

Perhaps five patients out of one hundred have this gift. It's a physical gift, in my opinion, and has little or nothing to do with education, relaxation techniques, or motivation, although those things alleviate fear. These women generally are close to delivery when they are admitted. In fact, some never make it to the hospital. Some give birth at home in the toilet because they thought they were having a hard bowel movement. The ones that make it to the hospital usually get an unneeded anesthetic.

The problem on admission is that most look like they are in pain. They are feeling a lot of intermittent pelvic pressure, which has been increasing in strength, frequency, and duration, and they are afraid of what is to come. Most get a quick, unnecessary anesthetic. But if you ask, "Are you in pain?" many will say something like, "No, it doesn't hurt now but it's going to, isn't it?" The response should be, "No, not for you it isn't, because you have this special gift!"

The other end of the spectrum is illustrated by a nurse patient of mine in my private practice. She worked in labor and delivery and had circulated on many of my deliveries. She knew that I liked to do natural childbirth and had heard me encourage selected patients to try it. She taught natural childbirth classes. She had a loving, attentive husband who was trained to be her labor coach. She had everything going for her.

When I entered the labor room to do her initial exam she was clutching the sides of the mattress with both hands. Her face was beet red and she was perspiring profusely. She groaned and said, "Oh, my God, I never knew anything could hurt so badly." She was in good labor but was barely dilated. She had a long way to go. It's a physical gift and she didn't have it. She really enjoyed her epidural.

After years of experience and observing and listening to my patients, it seems that a woman's ability to tolerate labor is a spectrum. As mentioned, 5 percent or so have no pain. Another 35 percent or so have little enough pain that with education and training in natural childbirth techniques, confidence in their supportive doctor and nurses and, most of all, strong motivation, can enjoy the unmedicated experience. And it's well worth the effort because they feel an enormous sense of pride and accomplishment and believe they have done their very best for their baby. The other 60 percent hurt like hell, but a good epidural makes them all like the 5 percent.

During my entire career, I tried to avoid doing unnecessary procedures to my patients. If a patient gets in trouble while undergoing an indicated procedure, it's one thing. If trouble occurs while undergoing an unindicated procedure, it's quite another. So did I deliver 40 percent of my patients with natural childbirth? No. How about 5 percent? Not even close. The problem is, it's really hard to talk a woman in labor out of an epidural. Please believe that I really tried.

My patient Maureen illustrates the difficulty. I delivered three babies for her, all between 2 a.m. and 6 a.m. After she rolled by the labor desk for her first with me, one of the nurses said, "She's not in labor."

"No," I said, "it doesn't look like it."

But she had told me on the phone that she was having contractions lasting almost a minute every three minutes. She was smiling and cheerful and dressed to the nines, beautifully coiffed, made up and perfumed. She was like this for all of her deliveries.

The exam revealed that she was seven centimeters dilated, in advanced labor. When told, she smiled and said, "Oh, good, then I can have an epidural."

I said, "You don't need an epidural. It would be a sin to give you one."

I explained about "the gift" and told her that she would love having the baby by natural childbirth. Her response was, "Doctor, I drove forty miles one way for all my office visits because you and your group are the only doctors using epidurals. I want an epidural!"

One of my inviolable rules is: never hassle or give any grief to a woman in labor. So I gave her an epidural. At the six-week checkup, we again discussed this.

The second was more or less a repeat. 3 a.m., looking like she was at the Captain's Ball and causing me to think as I checked her, If you have to work at 3 a.m., this is the way to go.

She insisted on another epidural. At her six-week checkup she asked me, "Doctor, is it harder for you to do a delivery if your patient has an epidural?"

"Oh, no," I responded, "it's much easier. With natural childbirth I have to be very gentle and deliberate, as well as explaining what I am doing and what the patient will feel. It takes a lot more time."

"I just wondered," she said.

The same scenario played out with the third. Eight centimeters dilated, with that big smile, she anticipated her epidural. I started to try one more time to talk her out of it. She held up her hand and said, "Doctor, stop! You told me it is easier for you to do a delivery if your patient has an epidural and I'm telling you it's easier for me, so just give it to me without the propaganda." Alas, another unindicated procedure.

Another patient traveled a long way to our office for her pregnancy visits because we gave epidurals, and she did so because she wanted to watch her delivery. Her first baby was delivered under general anesthesia and she first remembered seeing the baby in her postpartum room, hours after the delivery. With the second, she asked for a spinal so she could watch her baby deliver, in the mirror that hung over the end of the delivery table. She got her spinal but she had required so much pain medicine during labor that she couldn't keep her eyes open to watch.

Epidurals are a little flakey and sometimes do not give complete numbness. In fact, I preferred to dose as lightly as I could so that the patient might feel a little pressure and be able to push the baby's head out themselves, rather than have me pull it out with forceps. This gave them the feeling of accomplishment that natural childbirth patients had and avoided the scary feeling some got when they saw obstetric forceps. But patients varied in their sensitivity to anesthetics and this patient was very sensitive and was completely numb for the delivery. Because of that, the delivery wasn't on the delivery table with the mirror. We rolled her into the delivery room in her labor bed and pulled back the sheet to move her onto the table—and there was the baby's head coming out. I completed the delivery easily as she looked at the ceiling and said, "Damn, missed another one." I felt terrible.

Then there is the hyper-motivated patient at the opposite end of the spectrum; the one that really needs an epidural but won't take it because she is determined to have natural childbirth. We'll call her Erin, and she provided me with one of the worst nights of my professional career.

Admitted for her first labor and accompanied by her sister, a nurse and childbirth class instructor who seemed to believe that any woman can do natural childbirth if she is motivated and properly taught, Erin screamed with every contraction. She screamed at the top of her lungs. I offered her, no, I begged her to let me give her an epidural. She and her sister vehemently refused and became very angry when I later repeated my desire to intervene. Erin said that the contractions were incredibly painful but that screaming distracted her and helped her cope. Well, they certainly distracted me; in fact they distracted all the doctors, nurses, and the other patients in the department, if not the entire hospital.

It was not a short labor. Back on one of the call room beds, my head buried in a pillow, I still heard every scream. Finally her sister called to say that she was ready for delivery. Was she ever ready! The baby's head was crowning way out, and Erin desperately needed an episiotomy to let her deliver. The only problem, nurse sister didn't want her to have one. It is true that many women can deliver a baby without needing an episiotomy, but it was obvious that Erin was going to tear badly if the incision to enlarge the vaginal opening wasn't made. As I leaned in from the right side of the labor bed, scissors in hand, sister leaned in from the left side and pushed me away with her shoulder. With a loud pop, Erin's bottom literally exploded.

After handing off the baby—who was fine—I delivered the placenta and inspected the damage. It was a complete perineal tear, a devastating injury, the only one I ever had to deal with.

This tear, actually twin lacerations, which extended up the vagina from both sides of the opening and downward and backward on each side of the rectum, were deep, extending through the muscular sling (levator ani) that supported the pelvic and abdominal contents. There was much bleeding requiring immediate clamping and tying of numerous blood vessels followed by a move to the operating room for the repair. Erin didn't want to be put to sleep, or get a spinal, and asked me to repair it under local anesthesia—anything to make things more difficult. The repair took over two hours, and this in the wee hours of the morning.

When flesh tears, it does not do so evenly but jaggedly. When a muscle tears completely, it retracts and can be difficult to find, as the surrounding tissue covers it and blood colors everything the same. I had concerns that her bladder and bowel function might be compromised because these muscles supported those organs and because nerves were also torn. I meticulously searched out every layer, matched it with the other side, and sewed them back together with many stitches. How many? I couldn't count that high!

Erin did very well post-operatively. She was not a complainer and—despite all the screaming she did in labor—she seemed to have a high pain threshold. At the six-week checkup, the results were unbelievable. The scars were barely visible and her bottom looked normal with no hollows, lumps, or divots. Her bowel and bladder function was normal and she had no complaints. I attributed this mostly to her superior protoplasm as she was in excellent health, well nourished and in great shape at the end of her pregnancy. I did, however, feel good about my repair.

At her next annual checkup, Erin told me of her plans to have another baby—in fact, she was already trying to get pregnant. We had a long discussion. Though I cherished her as a patient, I told her that if I took care of her again I would insist that she take an epidural and have an episiotomy. I explained that scars tend to be brittle and that the likelihood of another tear was high and even though she had a perfect result she might not be so lucky the next time.

She left me and went to another doctor and delivered her second baby at another hospital. Sometime later I learned that she did natural childbirth, without an episiotomy and didn't tear. Shows how much I know!

CHAPTER THREE

Cesarean Sections and VBACs: Two's a Charm

~~~

My favorite new obstetric patient was the one who first came to me with her second pregnancy. It was as though I could do no wrong. No matter how I performed, she would almost certainly like it better than her first. (Erin was a good example, but one whom I didn't benefit from.) Being able to give epidurals to patients who had their first baby elsewhere, however, provided many opportunities for extra credit.

A twenty-four-hour labor with a two-hour second stage (pushing with every contraction) is not unusual with the first baby. Even if the second baby is bigger and weighs a pound or so more, the process is almost always quicker and easier. If the patient gets her first epidural with the second baby, she tends to give the epidural and the doctor too much credit, and I never minded that.

Most women will say that their third baby was harder to have than their second. That, I think, is a fault of their memory.

Because of the vast difference between the first two, they recall the second labor and delivery as being even easier than it actually was. They have forgotten how quickly the contractions got really hard and how close together they were.

These days, many women are delivered by caesarean section; the rate nationally is over 30 percent. Most, in my opinion, are unnecessary. It should be between 10 and 20 percent, and I achieved that rate managing a high-risk residents' clinic, as well as my own private practice. A recent study of Amish patients showed excellent results with a 6 percent section rate. To achieve low rates, the obstetrician must be expert at evaluating labor, maintaining fetal well-being, and the use of forceps and vaginal breech deliveries; in other words, be properly trained and have the self-confidence and judgment to provide the patient with effective, safe, and cost-effective care. In our litigious society it does take guts to practice cost-effective medicine, but it can and should be done. Many obstetricians that I knew practiced this way and never had a bad result and never got sued.

A vaginal birth after a caesarean section (VBAC) is very desirable because it is better and much more gratifying for the patient and is more cost-effective. A large percentage of c-sections are repeats, and 80 percent of these will have—and should have—easy vaginal deliveries. Easy because that is the only kind you let them have. For if any problem occurs in labor, the doctor simply performs a c-section.

Of course, if there is a persistent indication such as a pelvic outlet not big enough to deliver a baseball, let alone a baby's head, or any reason to believe that healing of the uterine incision was not adequate, then that patient is not a candidate and should be scheduled for a repeat section. The vast majority, however, are good candidates. Very few VBACs are being done, though, for two main reasons.

The first is the increased input required by the obstetrician and the malpractice issue if things are mishandled and/or damage to baby or mother occurs. The solution for the obstetrician: be in attendance during the labor or have a qualified substitute in your place, and do it right. VBACs generally don't take a long time. This is not the first baby, so labor is going to be more efficient and faster. If it isn't, resolve the problem easily and quickly, or do a repeat caesarean.

The second reason is the difficulty in talking the patient into doing it. Many of these women have very bad memories of their first labor—long and hard and after hours of effort, sometimes even with two or three hours of pushing, and in the end fruitless. Their best memory is the caesarean. They need to know that the doctor allows only one hard labor, that they've already had theirs, and that the success rate for having a vaginal birth is 80 percent. Their recovery time is much shorter, and their sense of achievement is very great.

My patients didn't get much of a choice. If I wasn't persuasive enough, I scheduled their repeat caesarean a little late to allow them to start labor, met them on admission, and addressed their reluctance again. One patient was so fearful that she wrote me a three-page letter detailing her fears and begging me not to make her labor. I thought that this might be a psychiatric indication for a scheduled repeat caesarian but dismissed that idea. I met her at the hospital; she was not very uncomfortable but was already six centimeters dilated, with the fetal head well down. After a quick epidural she was eight centimeters dilated and happy with the process. She and her husband watched the delivery, which was very easy and beautiful, and they were thrilled beyond words. She then wrote me a five-page letter telling me about it and how much she loved me for making her do it.

At her six-week checkup, she was still going on about how wonderful the experience was. She told me that although she and her husband only wanted two children, they had enjoyed that birth so much that they had decided to have another baby to relive it. This was a red flag to me. I told her about third deliveries and how unlikely that it would be as good as the second. There were no guarantees, I said. She was not hearing it.

In a few months, she was pregnant. Two weeks before her due date she called when her water broke. On admission the baby was crossways (transverse lie) with the umbilical cord presenting, and an immediate, emergency caesarean was done. Mother and baby did well, but in the ensuing weeks I spent a lot of time talking to her to help her get over her postpartum depression.

CHAPTER FOUR

Messy and Blue: Depression, Too

Delivering a baby provides the doctor with a teachable moment. The mother and father are a captive audience and, especially with the first baby, eager to learn. It's also a great time to build rapport with patients and to dispel fears before they arise. The teaching of personal and communications skills in residency training is now one of six basic competencies that must be acquired by the end of the four-year training program. Throughout this narrative I cover information that seemed to help patients and their husbands.

First, some examples of unhelpful communications: one of my chief residents was delivering the first baby of a clinic patient whom I had delivered seventeen years earlier. Her mother, still my patient, was in the delivery room and related the following to me. Her daughter, doing natural childbirth, was about to deliver, pushing with each contraction. With one push she uttered a soft, squealing grunt. The resident doctor said sternly, "We'll have no more of that."

The fetal head was about to deliver when the doctor realized that he had not provided enough room with his episiotomy and she was about to tear. He ordered her—too late—to stop pushing, something no woman would be able to do at that point. She delivered a healthy baby somewhat precipitously. The doctor then exclaimed, "Now look what you have done. You've blown out your bottom!"

At morning rounds the next day, I told my sixteen residents—including that resident—how one of them had conducted a delivery the day before. The residents were shocked and upset. One resident, a rather egotistical man, jumped up and said, "Dr. Rock, you have to tell them that wasn't me, because that's what they are all thinking." I did so and continued, "The patient's mother asked me to tell you something that she thinks you all need to know: a woman remembers her first labor and delivery in exquisite detail and never tires of telling everyone who will listen all about it and will do so for the rest of her life." Later, in my office, the offender received a severe reprimand and was sanctioned.

The second example involved the obstetrician covering my practice when I went out of town. I had chosen this individual because I so admired his intelligence and knowledge of the specialty, his technical expertise, and especially his dedication to exemplary ethics and morality. He was much admired by our colleagues and the nurses.

Just before leaving on a vacation, I was explaining to a patient who was almost due about my coverage. I told her how good Dr. Autry was and related the above to her but also told her that he didn't talk very much, and she would have to ask him questions to draw him out. My nurse began to laugh. "What's so funny?" I asked. "You don't remember," she said, "but you were away for my first delivery and Dr. Autry delivered me. When the baby came out, the umbilical cord flopped between its legs, and my husband said, 'It's a boy.' Dr. Autry held her up and chuckled and said, 'No, it isn't. It's a girl.' If my husband had not mistaken the sex, Dr. Autry would have come into the delivery room, delivered the baby, sewed me up, and left without saying a word. Those were the only words he said. He is really quiet!"

My medical school curriculum was heavy in psychiatry. At the time, most of my classmates and I thought it was a waste. We cut class a lot and went bowling at the local alley that gave students a big discount. I got my average up to 180. Once I was in practice, though, I realized that what I had learned in psych class about depression was invaluable and enabled me to help many, many patients. To try to head off postpartum depression, I usually started in the delivery room.

As a second-year medical student, I had learned from my wife after our first baby (a girl) that she had a lot of guilt because she thought our baby was really ugly. She told me she was glad I was going to be a doctor so we would be able to afford plastic surgery. Years later, in residency, I learned from my patients that many first mothers feel this way. It's really not too surprising because first babies are ugly, at least if they are the usual head-first variety, and they are really messy and blue until they get their first few breaths and are cleaned up.

The heads of first babies generally drop into the mother's pelvis three weeks or so before labor. This gives the mother more room under her ribs and is referred to as "lightening." With this, of course, the woman does notice increasing pelvic pressure. The fetal head is now ever more tightly confined in a tubular bony space that has no padding. If the pregnancy lasts full term, the head is always misshaped and lopsided and sometimes, depending on the position, severely so. If the back of the fetal head is toward the mother's back (posterior position) the head will be elongated, appearing as a "banana head." The nose is then mashed against the back of the mother's pubic bone and usually displaced to one side. If this first mother has never seen a brand new first baby, she has no idea that this is normal, and that in just a few days the head will round out, the nose will straighten, and her baby will be beautiful. In the delivery room, all she hears from the nurses and doctors who see through all the temporary deformities is how beautiful the baby is. I came to believe the guilt that mothers feel over this can be the start of a postpartum depression.

In subsequent pregnancies, the fetal head does not enter the pelvis early and the distortion is not nearly as great. Breech babies have beautiful heads from the get-go. At first, however, they all are messy and blue. My poor wife didn't know any of this. She was given a general anesthetic and her first remembered view of our little girl was when the nurse brought her into her postpartum room. She was shocked and disappointed, especially when the nurse brought in her roommate's baby, not her first, which was a really pretty little girl. The roommate was an indigent clinic patient, older and without a whole tooth in her head. My wife was sure there had been a mix-up of babies.

It became my routine to prepare first mothers and fathers while setting up for the delivery. I would ask, "Have you ever seen a brand new first baby?" I cheerfully told them that first babes are really ugly, and they are also messy and blue. Then I related the explanation above. When delivered, I held the baby up and commented on the distortions, pointing out how quickly their blue baby turned pink.

Guilt is the chief cause of depression, causing self-hate. The unprepared mother, hearing authority figures, the nurses and doctors, extol the baby's beauty, subconsciously feels that she is a bad person because she perceives the baby to be ugly. And there are many other opportunities later for a baby to cause the mother to feel guilty.

Whenever I saw a patient at her six-week checkup, I searched for signs of depression. The question a depressed person should ask themselves is, "Who do I hate that I love?" The big three for a new mother is the baby, the husband, or her mother—and sometimes it's all three. It is always someone whom she really loves. I never saw a patient depressed over having bad feelings toward her mother-in-law.

Not all babies are good babies. First babies, in particular, often don't sleep well, don't nurse well, and for weeks are simply incessantly demanding little blobs of protoplasm who give the mother no positive feedback whatsoever. Bad feelings toward the newborn well up, and upon inspection the mother can find no adequate reason for them. This is my baby, she thinks. How can I feel this way? The ultimate example was the mother who told me, as I explored her depression, that her baby was really bad, required nursing every two hours around the clock, and gave her no rest. After six weeks, she was completely exhausted when, one night, her baby nursed at 1 a.m. for about five minutes and fell asleep. She put the baby to bed and turned in herself, knowing that she would be up again at 3 a.m. As she drifted off to sleep, her last thought was, "Maybe he'll have a crib death and I'll be able to sleep." On that night, wouldn't you know, the baby slept through. She awoke at 6 a.m., leaped out of bed sure that her baby was dead. It was fine, but imagine the guilt she was saddled with.

I told this story to many patients, often before they went home from the hospital, or at the six-week checkup. As I related it to one new mother, she began crying. She had tears streaming down her face as I finished and she exclaimed, "My God, Dr. Rock, how can you know what's inside my head?" Apparently, it's in a lot of women's heads. Finding that they are normal and not bad mothers really helped these patients.

I once delivered a colleague's wife and apparently did not give her my talk before she went home. Her husband stopped in my office the day before his wife's six-week checkup to ask me to get his wife to see a psychiatrist. He told me that she was terribly depressed and couldn't care for the baby, didn't do anything, and stayed in bed much of the day. They had hired nurses around the clock. The next day I started to give her my depression talk. When I got to the part about bad feelings toward the baby she became very angry and insisted that she didn't have anything like that. She got up to leave. I ordered her to sit back down and listen to me. When I finished, she stormed out of the office. I thought, Man, you blew this friendship all to hell. Not so, it turned out. When I saw her husband a few days later he asked, "Eban, what did you say to my wife? She came home happy as a lark, whistling and energetic. She fired the nurses and is back to her old self." I said, "Oh, not much. I just convinced her that she wasn't a bad person."

Husbands are often worthy of a little hate. I saw this most often with career women who gave it up to have the baby—a woman who was used to being admired and respected for her abilities as a problem solver and for getting the job done. Now, suddenly she is stuck at home alone with this noncommunicating, incessantly demanding little being and it never stops! When hubby goes out the door in the morning to face another challenge and gain another victory she hates his guts. When he comes home and gives her an embrace, tells her how nice she looks, and proceeds to change baby's smelly diaper, and perhaps load the washer without being asked, the guilt hits. He is so wonderful, how can I feel this way? she thinks.

Mothers do it, too. For the new mother who is trying to nurse her baby fully, without supplemental bottles, to hear her mother repeatedly express doubt that the baby is getting enough may engender great irritation and perhaps a little hate.

So how can this guilt be headed off? The new mothers need to know that feelings are unasked-for-thoughts that pop into their heads, usually when they are most vulnerable.

These thoughts cannot be controlled any more than dreams can be controlled—and these feelings have no morality. They are just feelings. And there is always some justification for them. Newborns are demanding, without any consideration of the mother's fatigue. Husbands are sometimes unaware and unfeeling of their wife's inner turmoil, and wives' mothers can be a real pain in the patootie.

It really helps if the new mothers vent out loud. They need to hear themselves talking. To a bad baby, a mother can say in her sweetest voice—and with her most beatific smile—"Kid, you better let your mother sleep tonight or you might be out for the garbage man in the morning." Husbands are big boys and can be told, "You are a wonderful husband and I love you dearly, but when you walked out and left me with this child this morning I was hating your guts and hoping that you would drive off the bridge so I wouldn't have to look at your stupid face again."

How to deal with the grandmother I would leave up to them. When these kinds of feelings occur, a mother should tell herself, "That's a stupid feeling, and I'm just not going to think about it now. Maybe I will later but probably not."

Remember, most depression is caused by having bad feelings toward someone you really love, and feelings have no morality, and you can't control them.

So why feel guilty?

CHAPTER FIVE

Virgins I Have Known: Stretching the Truth

The petite Hawaiian rangerette conducted the group of fifteen tourists over the black lava field to a viewing platform. Five miles away Kilauea, in clear view, was fountaining bright red lava five hundred feet into the blue Hawaiian sky.

"I understand that in the past the natives would throw a virgin into the volcano as a sacrifice," a New Yorker said to the rangerette.

"They did, indeed," the young lady replied, "and there are very few of us left anymore."

Well, there are more than you might think. Virgins, in my experience, fly under the radar. Most don't advertise their status. Some are proud but extremely guarded and determined not to give it away until the perfect moment.

In my practice, in a very Roman Catholic part of town, I saw young ladies, brought in by their mothers, for premarital exams. In the 1960s and '70s, roughly 50 percent of this select group were virgins. I'm sure there are fewer now, but they are still out there.

So how do you tell? The short answer is, you can't, at least 99 percent of the time, you can't. Most hymens can admit most penises without tearing or over-stretching, especially these days when most girls have used tampons for several years before they have intercourse. Repeatedly withdrawing expanded tampons gently stretches the hymen to the point that initial sex is unlikely to be a traumatic event. So much for the examination by the Queen's gynecologist to certify the virginity of the woman betrothed to the prince.

At the other end of the spectrum, I do recall seeing a newly married patient after a year of infertility whose hymenal opening was so small that it barely admitted my little finger. She convincingly assured me that her husband was gaining full entry. A post-coital exam as part of the infertility workup showed a large pool of semen in her vagina, verifying that indeed he was. The best evidence of virginity is what the patient tells you, after you have defined the sacrosanct doctor-patient relationship and gained her confidence and trust.

Some of these virginal patients did have vaginal openings small enough to worry me that they might have a problem on their wedding night. So is a hymenotomy, the surgical cutting of the hymen, indicated? Never! The only indication for this is a completely imperforate hymen, with no opening at all. This impounds the menstrual flow, so the unfortunate child is brought to the doctor with monthly abdominal pain and no periods. In these rare cases, surgical incision under general anesthesia is indicated. Otherwise, hymenotomy should never be done, as it leaves scars that can remain tender long after healing. Gentle stretching does not leave such scars.

Hymens are very stretchable, and my partners and I offered to these women a "hymen stretch" as an office procedure. This had to be done a week or less prior to the wedding because, left alone for longer than that, the hymen would retighten. It's a simple and painless procedure involving the application of an anesthetic ointment, waiting five or ten minutes—we would do a ten-minute pregnancy visit in another room—then inserting a virginal vaginal speculum, which requires an opening about the width of a pencil. This would be opened while watching the patient's face until you saw a little wince. The instrument would then be held at that setting by tightening a set screw. After another few minutes—when enough room for a larger speculum was obtained—the process was repeated until there was judged to be room for normal intercourse. The whole process usually took less than an hour. I once stretched a hymen with an original opening that would just about admit the lead of a pencil.

Late one week I did a stretch on a bride-to-be and gave her my usual premarital "sex talk." Very early the next Sunday morning, my wife and I were awakened by the beep from the answering service. I briefly explained to my wife that this patient had just gotten married. She and her virgin husband (I discovered) were calling me from a nearby city, the first stop on their honeymoon.

"It isn't working," she said.

"It isn't working?" I repeated.

Wife became fully awake, listening. Thinking maybe vaginismus (involuntary vaginal spasm), which closes the vagina, I asked if he was able to get his penis in.

"Oh, yes," she said, "but nothing happens."

"Nothing happens?" I repeated.

Wife's face was now buried in her pillow.

"No," she said. "He says it feels like he's sticking it out the window."

I repeated that. Wife was gasping for breath. I had no idea where to go with this, so I asked to talk to her husband. He repeated the above. I was completely flummoxed!

"Well, um," I stammered, "usually with the warmth and tightness and the feeling you get with movement, things kind of happen automatically."

"Oh, you're supposed to move it?" he said.

My wife and I had a little trouble getting back to sleep. I saw the patient in the office three months later, nicely pregnant. She reported that everything was working fine.

Some years later, I attended a lecture by William Masters, MD, and Virginia Johnson of sexual research fame. I related this story to them. Dr. Masters told me that he had a very similar experience and was amazed at the anger expressed by the couple because he had not adequately explained the process to them.

The foregoing illustrates that virgins come in pairs and reminds me that I was once required to give telephone instructions to a virgin husband on how to deflower his virgin wife. A thirty-year-old attorney came in for a checkup and informed me that she was getting married. Oh, oh, I thought, because this woman was a bona fide virgin if there ever was one. She was one that had never been able to use tampons and required the tiny virginal speculum and still complained about discomfort with every exam. Raised in a very religious family and from a culture that had undoubtedly stressed the importance of virginity, she was also a setup for vaginismus.

I strongly recommended an office stretch procedure. She demurred. "I have had many friends," she said, "and they didn't have to do that."

"I'm sure that's true," I said, "but let me ask you a question. Has your fiancé ever touched or felt your breasts?"

"He wouldn't dare!" she indignantly exclaimed.

"Therein lies the problem," I said. "In most cases, when a couple reaches your station in life things have happened. Breasts have been bared and sucked on a bit; hands and fingers have explored each other's sex organs."

Her face contorted with disgust. "Fingers have felt into the vagina," I continued, "which gradually stretches the hymen so that intercourse without tearing can occur. Your hymen is very tight and on your wedding night, you are going to try to go from zero to sixty in a few seconds and it's not going to work very well."

She did schedule an appointment for the procedure a few days before the wedding, then called later and cancelled it.

I was very concerned and called her. She told me that she was sure that she and her husband could do it. I agreed that they probably would do all right but that he would have to be very slow and gentle and she would have to be able to relax her vaginal muscles adequately. I explained how those muscles work. "As you know," I told her, "women have three openings down there and they have muscles that control them. The rectum and bladder openings have doughnut-shaped muscles around them. The vagina has a hammock-like, sling-shaped muscle that keeps it closed. Those muscles are different from most of the body's muscles in that they have tone and are partially contracted all the time. This is why when you are sleeping and entirely relaxed you don't wet the bed. The muscles can be further tightened consciously or unconsciously when, for instance, you blow your nose. They can be completely relaxed consciously and also without one being aware that it is happening. This obviously occurs when you go to the bathroom and also when a woman really wants intercourse and does her part in making it occur. If the woman is afraid of pain, her vaginal sling muscles can contract more and actually go into spasm without her being aware of it (vaginismus). This pulls the outer third of the vagina up and almost behind the pubic bone, essentially closing the vagina. If you don't want pain and want to help your husband enter you, you have to learn to bear down and let the vagina go." She seemed to understand and thanked me.

Sunday noon, with my brother and two male friends in the car on the way to a professional football game, I got the call.

"We couldn't do it," she said.

I wasn't terribly surprised. I offered to meet them at my office after the game and do a stretch. She declined and asked, "Could you talk to my husband and tell him how to do it?"

Boy, would my passengers have loved that!

"Call me after 6 p.m." I said.

I had a little trouble concentrating on the game as I was composing the message in my head. That promised to be one long phone call.

When he called, I started by repeating the muscle story I had related to her. Then I told him, "Love her up and try to express your emotions as you tell her how much you love her. Show her how much you love her breasts and give them all the attention that she'll let you. Then feel her bottom and find her opening. You should do that with your little finger. Gently push it in. I suspect that she will tighten up and if you feel that happening stop pushing and tell her to bear down and let go, then push a little more. Whenever you feel her tighten anywhere during the process, stop and wait until she can relax her vagina. When you get your finger in—using the length of your finger, not the tip—gently pull toward her feet, encouraging her to bear down. Then sweep your finger from three o'clock to six to nine, to stretch things a little. If things go well, use your index finger the same way. Then use two fingers. If that works, look around for something a little bigger and put that in. You'll do fine. Good luck."

I waited a few weeks then called her. She reported that they were doing fine. It occurred to me later that I forgot to tell him to move it, but they must have figured that out. Another thought is that I should have billed for those long phone instructions as the pediatricians do, but I never did. If they would have asked me how much they owed me, though, I would have responded, "Oh, just pay me what it was worth to you."

CHAPTER SIX

Laparoscopy:
Seeing is Believing

After three years in private practice, my army reserve unit was activated. I had joined the reserves during my second year of residency so that I might avoid the Vietnam draft and finish my training. I had completed five years of the six-year obligation, attending all-day Sunday training sessions once or twice a month and five two-week summer camps. During my third year of private practice, with one year to go, Lyndon Johnson announced that to facilitate negotiations with the Vietcong he was ordering the cessation of the bombing of North Vietnam but—apparently to show our continued resolve—was activating selected army reserve units. My unit was one of the lucky ones. The call-up was for two years, but the units were all deactivated after a year.

My field hospital unit, staffed with twelve physicians, was eventually sent to Vietnam. Because of my specialty, I was assigned to Rader Army clinic at Fort Myer, Virginia, then to Dewitt Army Hospital at Fort Belvoir, Virginia. I was part of an ob/gyn staff that cared for mostly army dependent wives and female active-duty personnel. We also taught and supervised residents assigned there from Walter Reed Hospital.

I enjoyed teaching residents how to give epidurals, and do forceps and vaginal breech deliveries. In return, they introduced me to laparoscopy, a new procedure that had been recently utilized at Walter Reed. Initially, one could only look through the scope and view the pelvic and abdominal contents. The development of introducing instruments—and being able to operate through the scope—came later. Nevertheless, it was a godsend to gynecologists. One of our problems in those days was in diagnosing ectopic pregnancies, those located in the fallopian tube instead of the uterus.

When a patient had pelvic pain and was overdue for a period, this diagnosis had to be given serious consideration. Rupture of a tubal pregnancy can result in massive internal bleeding, shock, and rapid demise, if not quickly treated. Keep in mind, those were the days before ultrasound, CAT scans, and even very usable pregnancy tests. If a pelvic exam was inconclusive, which many were, the patient was admitted to the hospital where blood was readied for transfusion, and she was observed and reexamined for several days until the diagnosis was ruled in or out. Being able to look at the fallopian tubes changed everything.

After a year in the army, my unit was deactivated and I returned to my practice. Eager to make available this new procedure, I presented requests for the equipment to the three hospitals where I did surgery. A few weeks later, I had the unenviable experience of introducing the procedure at the three hospitals. Unenviable because it was time-consuming and not easy to start a new procedure involving techniques and instruments unfamiliar to the nurses and technicians. The insufflation equipment to fill the patient's abdomen with carbon dioxide and maintain the proper pressure of the gas was completely new. Operating room nurses have always been a select breed, however, and they quickly understood the value of the procedure, and they easily became proficient.

One anesthesiologist did give me trouble. His name was McNanny, but the surgeons called him "McNasty" because he was quickly on their case if they were not performing to his expectations. The fact that he was perhaps the best anesthesiologist at this very large hospital allowed him to be that way without causing surgeons—in effect his referring physicians—to take their patients elsewhere.

My patient was a perfect candidate for the procedure. I had seen her in the office and she gave the typical history for a tubal ectopic pregnancy. The pelvic exam revealed tenderness in the area of the right tube but not signs of an acute abdomen, which would have indicated internal bleeding. So I thought that she probably didn't have an ectopic pregnancy, but I had to hospitalize her because I was unsure. I scheduled her for laparoscopy at 1 p.m. the next afternoon.

I arrived early to help the nurses assemble the unfamiliar equipment and explain its operation. Dr. McNanny showed up and soon was on my case, complaining about the slow pace and the procedure that he felt was ridiculous.

"Godammit, Rock, why don't you just make a little incision and look in there so we can get this done and get out of here?"

"Mac," I said, "I don't think that she has an ectopic, but I'm afraid to send her home. If I can see both tubes and rule it out, she will go home this evening without pain instead of having lots of post-op pain and four or five days in the hospital."

"Oh, bullshit," he exclaimed, "I don't believe that for a second. You young guys just have to find new things to screw around with."

The procedure, though slow, went well and I could see both tubes well and ruled out the tubal pregnancy. From the recovery room, my patient was taken back to her room, which was a five-bed open ward. I paid her a visit about 4:30 p.m. I mentioned that she was the perfect patient for the procedure and she was, in more ways than one. She was a beautiful twenty-one-year-old blonde with hair down to her waist and a lovely figure. She was sitting on the edge of her bed in a sheer nightgown and playing her guitar and singing to the other four women in the room. The late winter sun was streaming through the window illuminating her. She was happy to see me and told me that she had had some upper chest and shoulder discomfort for a while but it had gone away. (I figured out later how to prevent that.)

She was very happy that the new procedure was used and told me that her family was on the way to take her home. Everyone had been so nice to her, she said, "Especially the anesthetist (as she called Dr. McNanny)."

The little light bulb lurking invisibly over my head flashed on. "Why don't you ring the nurses' station after I leave and ask them to call down to surgery and see if Dr. McNanny will come up to see you?" I said. "I know it would make him happy to see how well you are doing."

An hour or so later, I visited her again. Her family had just arrived. "You just missed Dr. McNanny," she said. "He just left. He sat here for the longest time and had me sing him five or six songs. I think that he liked me."

"I'll bet he did," I replied.

A few days later I ran into McNanny in the doctor's dining room.

"Mac, what do you think of that new procedure?" I asked.

"Oh, Eban," he said enthusiastically, "I think it's going to work out. It seems like a real good procedure."

He never gave me any more trouble.

A year or so later, I greeted my patient and her husband by the bar at my son's wedding reception and discovered that she was the aunt of my new daughter-in-law. I enjoyed telling them the story of how she helped me whip a nasty anesthesiologist into shape.

The post-operative upper chest and shoulder pain experienced by laparoscoped patients caused me to think. As a scuba diver, I was aware of the solubility of carbon dioxide in blood, which is why we use it to inflate the abdomen and the relative insolubility of nitrogen, which constitutes 80 percent of air. A long tube of significant diameter conducted the carbon dioxide from the insufflator to the patient. That tubing held a lot of air, which was pushed into the patient's abdomen ahead of the carbon dioxide. In addition, at the end of the procedure during the removal of the sleeve through which the scope was introduced—and while closing the incision—it was very easy to let air get sucked into the abdomen. These things were all easy to eliminate.

Flushing the tube, needle or trocar with carbon dioxide eliminated the nitrogen. When removing the scope and sleeve, special care must be taken not to let air get sucked in. Instead of working so hard to get all of the carbon dioxide out of the abdomen, I left a little in. This, because of its solubility, will be rapidly absorbed. If some bubbles came out during the closure, that's great, as it prevented air from going in. These precautions completely eliminated the post-op chest discomfort. The injection of a long-acting local anesthetic to the incision site of the anesthetized patient five minutes before making the incision eliminated post-op incision pain, and the patients awakened with no pain at all.

The head nurse of the hospital's post-surgery recovery unit was my patient and asked me to do a laparoscopic tubal ligation on her. She mentioned her concern about the post-op chest pain she had seen many patients suffer. All of my laparoscopic patients were done in the out-patient unit, and she was not familiar with what I was doing. I explained it to her and she was totally unbelieving. She was back to work the day after her procedure and came up to my office to give me a box of premium chocolates. She reported that the only way she could tell anything was done to her was the scratchy throat she had from the endotracheal tube.

CHAPTER SEVEN

Shock and Awe: Mrs. Doe Fends For Herself

My patients never turned out to be anything like the initial impression they gave me. The best example of that was Nan, a twenty-four-year-old with a beautiful face and figure. Her blonde hair was pulled back into a bun and she wore stylish glasses. That, combined with her perfect posture and precise manner of speaking—each word perfectly enunciated—gave me an impression of sophistication and a bit of prudishness. I was on my best professional behavior.

As usual, I took a complete history and did a complete physical exam. I then went to the lab to check vaginal smear slides while the patient got dressed. At the last talk, as my nurses called it, we discussed Nan's efforts to get pregnant. They had stopped using contraception six months before. I reassured her by telling her that in couples with normal fertility, it can take up to a year.

I reviewed her history and noted that she was a teacher. I asked her what grade she taught. "Eighth grade," she replied.

Oh, oh, I thought, as I looked at her and asked, "Eighth-grade boys?"

Eighth-grade boys are bundles of raging hormones and I knew there would be an issue.

"Yes, Doctor," she replied.

"Oh, my goodness," I said. "I'll bet they give you fits."

"They do, indeed," she replied. "Just yesterday, for example, I was passing out tests that I had graded and noticed something written on an empty desktop. I really get upset when students deface their desks. I leaned over and read, 'I'd like to suck Mrs. Doe's tits.'"

After I picked myself up off the floor, I said, "I'm so sorry. That had to be terribly difficult for you. What did you do?"

"I straightened up and looked around and asked, 'All right, which one of you little mothers wrote that?'"

Off my chair again! She was tough as nails, as she had to be to handle eighth-grade boys.

A year later Nan returned and requested that we start an infertility workup, as they had been unsuccessful in their quest. She had always had irregular cycles, four to sometimes seven weeks apart, but basal body temperatures revealed that she was ovulating and had a good post-ovulatory temperature rise. Her husband's sperm count was devastating, however, showing zero sperm. This is untreatable, and I discussed donor insemination or adoption. She demurred, and at her next checkup a year later, she informed me that they had divorced.

Another year passed, and at her annual checkup she was six weeks from her last period, nothing unusual for her. Upon her pelvic exam I noticed that her uterus, instead of feeling like a flattened pear about the size of a man's thumb—usual in a patient that has never been pregnant—felt like a rounded pear and was very soft. I caught my nurse's eye, then glanced at Nan's urine sample on the counter. When I entered the lab, the nurse was already running the pregnancy test. It was very positive.

I did not want to tell Nan. "This poor woman," I said to my nurse. "She wanted to be pregnant so badly and even ended up getting divorced over it. Now she is pregnant and isn't even married. I don't want to tell her this. You tell her," I said to the nurse.

"You're the doctor," my nurse said. "You have to tell her."

Back to the exam room I went.

"I don't know how to tell you this," I said, "but, Nan, you are pregnant."

"Are you sure?" she asked.

"Yes," I said. "Your uterus is enlarged and your pregnancy test is very positive."

"Good," she responded. "Now I'll marry him."

Sadly for me, after a couple of pregnancy visits her new husband's employer transferred him across the country, and I never saw her again.

Another patient shocked me at a post-surgical checkup. I had done some vaginal surgery on her, as I recall, a vaginal hysterectomy four weeks previously. The vaginal cuff was well-healed and she was feeling great. After checking her vaginal flora (microscopic bacteria), I returned to the exam room to report to her and her husband. He was seated on the low stool I had sat on to inspect her vaginal incision. The patient and I were seated at the small wall desk.

"Doctor, is it all right if we have sex?" she asked.

"I believe so," I replied, "but you'll have to go easy for a while."

I turned to the husband and said, "Maybe use only half of it for a couple of weeks or so."

"Half of it," The patient vigorously retorted, "he only has this much." And she held her thumb and forefinger about two inches apart.

The poor husband looked up at me with the most pathetic look and said, "Oh, Doc, she does this stuff to me all the time."

Another real shocker came from a pediatrician and occurred because I violated one of my cardinal rules. The rule was to immediately tell the patient of any abnormality of the baby.

"We have a little problem," I would say, then I showed the parents the cleft lip or the birthmark, and I continued on about how it could be fixed. Of course, not all things could be fixed.

While covering for the department chairman, I delivered his patient of her second baby and realized immediately that it was a Down Syndrome baby. Faced with the unpleasant task of telling her, I blinked. My rationalization was that she already had a very good pediatrician whom she knew well, whereas she had just met me. I decided that her pediatrician could do a much better job of explaining how to cope with this difficult problem. Then on rounds the next day, before I saw her, an agitated head nurse said to me, "He didn't tell her!"

I couldn't believe it. She went on to explain, "He said that every new mother deserves a few days of happiness before you lay on her this lifelong disability." I paced around the nurses' station for some minutes, regretting not having told her. Finally, I went to see her. She told me that the pediatrician had checked the baby and said that he was fine.

"Mrs. Smith," I said, "the baby is doing fine, but there is a serious problem." And I told her. She cried, of course, and said, "I knew something was wrong, because the nurses were acting so strange when they brought the baby out to me and when they came to take it back to the nursery."

That illustrated just one of the problems occurring when doctors and nurses are not on the same page. Her obstetrician returned the next day and resumed her care.

Some six weeks later, while going through my stack of mail, I found a letter from the pediatrician. He took me to task for telling her of the abnormality, stating his belief that I had deprived her of at least a few days of happiness and chided me for interfering with his relationship with the patient. The next piece of mail in the stack was a beautiful card from the mother. She thanked me for my care and especially for telling her the truth about the baby. She wrote that the baby was doing fine and that she had enrolled in a support group and was very happy and optimistic about their future.

I mentioned that her pediatrician was very good and he was. He had cared for a number of babies I had delivered, and until this episode, I was always happy when one of my patients chose him to care for their baby. So I wrote him a letter. I told him that I couldn't disagree more with his approach. I pointed out the difficulty it caused with the nurses. Then I wrote, "You know, sometime this mother is going to bring her sick, feverish child to you, and you are going to diagnose a URI (common cold) and assure her it is not serious, and she is not going to believe you because she knows that you do not always tell the truth."

Four or five years later at a restaurant in another city, I was approached by a petite blonde who asked, "Are you Dr. Rock?"

It was Mrs. Smith. She again thanked me and beamingly told me at length how well her baby was doing.

"He is going to be very teachable," she said, "and we're going to make him self-sufficient."

CHAPTER EIGHT

The Menstrual Cycle: Who's Got Rhythm?

Entering private practice in a very Roman Catholic part of town provided some unusual challenges. In those days, most Catholic women did not believe that they should use artificial contraception. The church declared it to be sinful and promoted the rhythm system as the only acceptable method. The basal body temperature method was said to be the most effective. My senior partner had perfected a method to help patients successfully practice what he called 100 percent effective rhythm. Of course, it was only 100 percent effective if couples could follow the rules.

By then, we were the parents of five of our six children, several conceived while "practicing" rhythm, although not following my senior partner's strict rules. Nevertheless, I joined my partners in helping patients with this system. I learned many things and verified discoveries about the physiology of reproduction that he had made and—to this day—are unknown or unaccepted by the medical community.

When I completed my residency in the mid 1960s, the lifespan of sperm in a woman's body after intercourse was said to be twenty-four to forty-eight hours. When the subspecialty of reproductive endocrinology and infertility developed, studies showed that it was more like forty-eight to seventy-two hours, which is still accepted as accurate.

Would you believe fourteen days? As is well known, women ovulate near mid-cycle, day fourteen of a "normal" twenty-eight-day cycle (actually it's fourteen days before the next period). A woman's basal body temperature (bbt), the lowest temperature attained each twenty-four hours, occurs during the early morning hours after she has been asleep for at least four to six hours and persists until she is up and about for several minutes in the morning. Before ovulation, from cycle day two or so, until after ovulation, the temperature is always below 98 degrees, usually in the high 96 to 97.5 range. Of course, a fever or certain medical illnesses (hyperthyroidism) can negate that.

Heavy alcohol intake or very restless sleep will somewhat affect the bbt. On the day of, or within a day or two after ovulation, the bbt will begin to rise to above 98 degrees, sometimes abruptly, but more often spread over a few days. The elevation persists until just before or during the first few days of the menstrual period. If pregnancy occurs, the bbt goes higher, often near 99 degrees, and stays there for at least, the first three months. This is so reliable that a bbt of over 98 for twenty-one days from the documented rise after ovulation, without fail, indicates pregnancy. If it continues to rise to the high 98s, it indicates a normally growing pregnancy, in contrast to a falling temperature, which indicates an inevitable spontaneous abortion (medical term for miscarriage).

The temperature rise after ovulation occurs because the follicle in the ovary that produced the egg (corpus leuteum) persists for a while as a hormone-producing organ and releases increasing amounts of progesterone, which is thermogenic, into the blood stream. Once the progesterone level reaches a certain point, which seemed to be after three days of elevated temperatures, it blocks other follicles from ovulating. It's interesting that a mature woman has about four hundred thousand follicles in her ovaries but can only ovulate about 480 eggs in her lifetime (forty years times twelve a year). Many follicles start to ripen each cycle, but the first one or two (a tie that can result in fraternal twins) block the rest and they dry up. This then, is the basis for the bbt rhythm system.

We supplied our patients with bbt charts and instructions on how to take and chart their bbt. The temperature must be taken by 7 a.m., before getting out of bed. Notations about alcohol intake or restlessness should be made. If intercourse occurred, the temperature dot on the chart was circled. At mid-cycle, the patient called the office and gave the nurse the temperatures, then the nurse created a duplicate bbt chart and informed the patient as to when the doctor would call.

At call back, the doctor interpreted the bbt graph for the patient. The patients appreciated this because, as one patient told me, "It's hard to read your temperature graph correctly when you're horny."

Calls went like this:

"Mrs. Smith, you're safe today."

"Mrs. Jones, you're not safe but if your temperature is as high tomorrow as it is today, you will be safe. If not call the office."

"Mrs. Doe, you're not safe; call in around three days with more temperatures."

The interpretation was then noted on the graph.

Day in and day out, at the end of office hours, two doctors interpreted fifteen to thirty bbt charts each. We had a system for this. Two nurses used eight phone lines to call the patients and put them on hold, then wrote the number of phone line above the latest temperature. Then they passed the chart to the doctor. The conversations, as noted above, were usually very brief. For this service we charged $10 annually. I did this for nine years, reviewing thousands of bbt graphs. Some of our colleagues claimed that we controlled the sex lives of most of the western side of town. When told this, my senior partner said indignantly, "We do not tell them when to have sex. We tell them when they are safe."

It's difficult to believe these days that so many women used this method. These women were religious and believed that this was the only acceptable method. The number using this did gradually fall, as more Catholic women found birth control pills to be acceptable.

There were two major problems with the method, once you got past the effort required to take and chart the temperature every day. The first had to do with the lifespan of sperm. My partners had quickly noted, and I verified, that patients were getting pregnant from intercourse as much as two weeks before ovulation. This wasn't common but happened often enough to verify that, in very fertile couples, sperm can survive for that length of time and still fertilize the egg.

The patient that best convinced me of this showed up in my office pregnant, with chart in hand. It showed that the last intercourse was on the third day of her period. That was because her husband had left that day for three weeks in Japan. Her bbt chart clearly showed that she had ovulated on the sixteenth cycle day when her bbt rose to 98. Her husband returned on the twenty-fourth cycle day, as her temperature rose to 98.8 and stayed there. Her pregnancy went well and her delivery date correlated with conception at the time that her temperature rise had occurred. When I discussed this with my colleagues in other practices, they of course said that the baby was likely not her husband's. I knew better. I knew her well and was positive that it could only be their baby. I also knew that were it otherwise, with the relationship we had developed, she would have told me.

How can this be? When semen is deposited in the vagina, the sperm have at best a few hours to get out of the vagina and into the cervix. The secretions in the vagina are acidic and very hostile to sperm. Semen is very alkaline and neutralizes the acid for a few hours. Many sperm enter the cervical canal, which is alkaline and glucose rich—a very hospitable environment for them. Most quickly swim up the canal, through the uterus and out the tubes, perhaps added by muscular contractions of those organs. If there is no egg present and ready for fertilization at the ovary, they are lost in the pelvic cavity and are absorbed. Some apparently get sidetracked and end up in the cervical mucus glands. These long, tortuous, tubular glands provide the suitable secretions in the cervix. There, the sperm can bump around for various amounts of time until they get back out into the canal where they again head north. If this is true, then the ovaries are being seeded with sperm in decreasing numbers for up to fourteen days. This hypothesis would be very difficult to prove, requiring an invasive procedure to collect mucus from these glands. I do recall that during my residency I heard about a small unpublished study where mucus was collected from fresh hysterectomy specimens. The investigator had asked patients to have a last unprotected intercourse at various intervals before their scheduled surgery and to use a condom after that. He reported finding live motile sperm in the glandular mucus two weeks after the last unprotected intercourse.

The rules then, for 100 percent effective rhythm, went like this. No sex from the second day of the menses until the bbt is elevated above 98 for three days—and the doctor must make that determination. Now, if a woman had a twenty-eight-day cycle, intercourse was safe, at most, from day seventeen to day two of the next cycle, a total of thirteen days. That's assuming that her bbt rose abruptly and stayed on a plateau the next three days, and few did. Most rose slowly over three or four days, and some never did plateau before their menses started.

Unworkable as it sounds, we did have many patients who apparently were able to successfully avoid pregnancy this way. Most, however, were taking chances and having sex up to the seventh to tenth cycle day. Life got easier by the late 1970s when many Catholic women decided that the use of oral contraceptives was permissible for them.

If sperm can fertilize up to two weeks post-intercourse, as I am convinced is true, think of the implications this has for barrier methods. Many couples start using condoms or their diaphragm "at ovulation time," as I was often told. A well-fitted diaphragm properly used, in my experience, is far better than the 98 percent effective usually touted. My diaphragm patients who got pregnant would often tell me "Yes" when I asked if they had used the diaphragm. But not being easily satisfied, I would then ask, "How about during the tail end of or just after a period, "Did you use it then?" Virtually all of those pregnant would say, "Oh, no. You can't get pregnant then. We start using it on the tenth (or so) cycle day." Method failure or patient failure—you be the judge.

The proper use of a diaphragm entails separating it from the lovemaking by making it part of the bathroom routine on the way to bed—like contact lenses in reverse. At night, you take out your contacts and put in the diaphragm (with contraceptive jelly but without thought of why). In the morning, take out the diaphragm and put in the contacts, and don't get them mixed up as you can't see well through a diaphragm. I had many patients who liked this method very much. One volunteered that its use improved their sex life, causing her to initiate lovemaking more often, instead of wasting the jelly. Husbands will love that effect and won't question the reason.

Another benefit of my patients keeping a bbt chart was that it gave me a few extra nights in my own bed. When one of those middle-of-the-night calls came with the patient complaining of sharp pain low on one side or the other, ectopic tubal pregnancy was always a big concern. I learned to ask these patients if they were keeping a chart. If so, I would have them read me the temperatures since the end of the last period. If they were low or just beginning to rise, I would know that they couldn't be pregnant and were likely to be ovulating, which can occasionally be quite painful (called mittelschmerz or mid-pain).

A little reassurance and back to sleep I went.

CHAPTER NINE

Women Are From Venus: Men Are From Elsewhere

〜

When I began private practice, joining a two-man group as a full partner on day one, my senior partner asked me if I knew how to do a non-directive psychiatric interview.

"Of course," I said.

He then gave me a few instructions. "You should talk to all of your new patients about sex," he said. "After taking a complete medical history, do a non-directive psychosexual interview. Start by asking them if they have any problems with sex and intercourse. Next, be sure to ask how frequently they have intercourse (to identify the undersexed male). If orgasm hasn't been mentioned by this time, ask them if they reach orgasm with intercourse. With each patient response, remain non-directive and ask things like, 'How do you feel about that,' or 'How does that make you feel?' Your patients will teach you what you need to know to enable you to counsel and advise those that have problems."

I learned a lot in a very short period of time because—in contrast to psychiatrists, psychologists, and sex counselors who see only patients with problems—I was interviewing seven to ten new patients a week, and most were normal women who had few or no problems with sex, or, at least, not enough to feel they needed help.

Women in their first few months of marriage really enlightened me. Several who answered "No" when asked about spontaneous orgasm with intercourse responded similarly to my question, "How do you feel about that?" The responses were best expressed by one patient who said, "It doesn't bother me a bit, but it sure bothers my husband."

Further conversations revealed that these women, even though they really wanted sex, were not thinking physical thoughts about what they were going to feel. It was an entirely emotional experience:

"He really needs me."

"He makes me feel beautiful."

"I can't believe how aroused I can make him."

"I love to satisfy him."

"When he is finished I feel really good—full of love."

But then some would say, "After a while, he started asking me if I came." One said, "I asked myself, is there supposed to be more?" She might have been related to the virgin husband discussed in Chapter Six.

These women were saying that even though they didn't achieve orgasm, they were completely satisfied. Wow! Women can do something that men can't even comprehend. They can want and have sexual intercourse and be totally satisfied without having an orgasm. It became apparent to me that women start off with a sex drive that is almost 100 percent emotional. This was confirmed for me when I questioned young, sexually active single women as to why they first decided to have sex. Some expressed curiosity about what it would be like, but some related that they wanted to satisfy their partner—that they were amazed by how badly he seemed to need them. Again, all emotional.

Most women do develop the physical need for intercourse and achieve physical satisfaction from it. This seems to occur more quickly if they don't try to force it to happen. The problem is that often their partner, who has heard the erroneous information that women are slower than men and require extended foreplay and more stimulation and prolonged intercourse, wants her to come, and begins to really work at it. I think he wants this in order to gain for him emotional satisfaction in knowing that he has satisfied this woman he loves. Working so hard sometimes causes physical problems for women, such as recurrent cystitis (bladder infections). Yes, ladies, men do need emotional sexual satisfaction. When they are young, it is a very secondary need, but it's there.

Foreplay sometimes seem to get a women into the physical mood that results in a spontaneous orgasm, but when I questioned women who told me this, they often recalled that earlier in the day they were aware that the physical need was there. It had just gotten lost in the cares of the day.

Listening to my patients also led me to believe that working to get an orgasm could decrease their emotional satisfaction.

When their man had a fast and apparently profound orgasm, the wife knew she was really good.

I inquired of a number of patients how they felt when they were first asked the dumb question, "Did you come?" Several reported confusion and disappointment and questioned themselves as to why he was asking. Some thought, "Wasn't I good enough for him?" Many women actually think, early on, that their partner can feel their orgasm with his penis. Here's news for you, girls. He can't. I believe also that a woman cannot feel a man's orgasm. There may be a few exceptions—one patient told me, "His penis throbs when he comes"—but from what I hear, if you can feel your partner's orgasm, you are a rare bird indeed.

Many women discover that their man cannot feel their orgasm when they resort to faking it, and they get away with it for a while. I never recommended this. There is an easier and more honest way. In this case, the best defense is a good offense. All a woman has to do is convince her man that she is completely satisfied, and he will assume that she has had an orgasm, and she can do this without lying. If a woman perceives that her husband needs her and knows that her mood is not physical, she can wait for it to play out, or she can initiate sex as she would do if she were physical, making it a better experience for both. Then if she tells him—before he asks—that she is satisfied, he will be fulfilled. It really helps if the satisfaction message is couched in physical terms. If she says what she thinks, it would likely be, "I love you so much." That might not get it. Changing a word or two will. "I loved it" has a different sound. "You really know what's good for me or how to satisfy me." "That was a good one." Or a simple heartfelt "thank you" would likely work well. There is his emotional satisfaction, and now he has it all.

I cautioned women against trying to explain to their lover that she really can be satisfied without reaching orgasm. To make a young man understand that her emotional orgasm is as good and satisfying as his physical orgasm is a tall task indeed. He will just start asking, "What kind was that one?" It's much easier and better to teach him.

One patient, after working on the above information for a year, said that she explained it to her husband as follows: "Sometimes I feel my orgasms more in my pelvis and sometimes more in my heart." That caused him to ask her, "Where was that one mostly?" (I should explain that individual patients gave me this kind of information in bits and pieces about a year apart, when they came in for their annual checkup.) She told me that she solved her problem by asking him back, "Why are you asking me that? I'm lying here completely satisfied and thinking that I was really good for you, and you make me think that I wasn't. Wasn't I?" Another said she got her husband to stop asking by responding in a very disappointed tone, "Honey, couldn't you tell?"

Now about the physical mood. The very most consistent answer I got when questioning young patients about sex was when I asked them how often their mood was physical, or how often they had a spontaneous orgasm with intercourse (same question). Over and over again I would hear, "once or twice a month" or "every two to four weeks." At first when I heard this, I was shocked. In my early thirties I thought, This is terrible; women need it twice a month and men want it every day. I asked the patient, "So you really, really only need sex once or twice a month?"

"Oh, no," she said emphatically, "if he didn't need me at least two or three times a week or more, I would feel unattractive, undesirable and insecure, and might start to worry that he was seeing someone else."

I learned a lot that day!

Over the years, I tried to relate that physical need to a woman's cycle, but answers were not very consistent. Many did say that it was often right after their period. It did become apparent that, as some woman get older, the frequency of physical mood increases to as often as once a week, or a little more. Most agreed that if they were in that mood, they had little or no need for foreplay, at least as the recipient of it. Women in the physical mood are a different kind of animal. They just want to get on with it. One patient told me that after one of these episodes her husband became emotional and began to tell her how much he loved and needed her, especially when she gave herself so completely to him like that.

"I didn't tell him, but I wasn't giving," she told me. "I was taking."

"What were you taking?" I asked.

She became thoughtful and finally said, "I was being completely selfish and taking my pleasure from him—not thinking of him at all."

A pretty wonderful thing sex is when, whether male or female, you can selfishly take pleasure from your lover and at the same time give you partner complete satisfaction.

This selfish, physical aspect gives some women trouble and perhaps causes them to be unable to achieve orgasm. Interviewing a patient whom I thought might have this problem, I asked, "Suppose that I made house calls and I walked in on you and your husband having intercourse and asked you, 'What are you doing?' How would you answer?"

"We're making love," she said.

"How would your husband answer?" I asked her.

She became pensive, colored a bit, and said, "Uh, he might say, 'We're having sex.' Or something worse," she added and really turned red.

In my medical school psychiatry classes, I learned that the subconscious mind has profound influence over how we function. If we are raised to think that sex is improper or wrong or dirty, it can cause problems, particularly in preventing spontaneous orgasm in women. As my reputation of talking to my patients about sex got around, I did begin to see some new patients with sexual pathology. Some of these I referred to mental health specialists gifted in sex counseling, but many more I was able to help by informing them of the possible mechanism of their problem and making suggestions on how to deal with it, as I did with patients who were depressed.

The patient discussed above was easy. I explained to her what I had learned about sexual physical mood in women and about subconscious inhibition, and I pointed out that if she found herself in the physical mood it would benefit her husband greatly if she could make herself be selfish and uninhibited. I explained that she may have to confront her subconscious mind and tell it that you don't care if it thinks it is unacceptable; you are going to do it anyway. You might accomplish this by hearing yourself tell your husband what you want him to do to you, using physical words such as slang terminology and, if you can, name parts of your anatomy that you would like him to pay particular attention to, but perhaps don't use the proper anatomic names for them. If you are really in the physical mood, you're probably thinking those things, anyway.

She appeared a little shell-shocked when she left, but a year later she told me that it worked. She went on to say that for a long time she had to hear herself say the F-word to have an orgasm, but more recently that wasn't always necessary.

This method worked well for a lot of patients, but there was one who returned after a year and told me that she was sure I was right when I told her that if she used words like that she would have an orgasm. She went on to tell me that making love to her husband was such a beautiful and precious thing, she was not going to debase it that way and decided that she didn't need to have a physical orgasm. Different strokes for different folks, I thought.

Another patient told me that her discussion with me had really helped because she could come much closer to reaching spontaneous orgasm with intercourse but couldn't quite get there. After she refused my efforts to refer her to a psychologist or psychiatrist, she returned for another checkup.

She wanted to talk again about her difficulty. I asked her to go through the sequence of events that always ended in failure. Listening to her, I was amazed to hear her say that she reached the point where she was thinking the slang word and would start to come. She suddenly stopped talking and got a distant look in her eyes, then proceeded to say, "I wonder what my mother would think of me if she knew what I was doing." That was revealing, indeed. The poor woman was taking her mother to bed with her. When, even with this discovery, she couldn't achieve orgasm, I again urged her see a professional counselor. I suspected that perhaps at this point she didn't love her husband and was subconsciously holding back to deprive him. Whatever it was, I didn't have enough training to continue. She refused again. Some months later, I discovered that she was having an extramarital affair, which soon led to a divorce. I regarded this as a failure on my part but still don't know what else I could have done.

Routinely discussing sex with my patients provided other benefits in that it caused them to be introspective between visits. Then they were able to tell me some incredible things they had discovered. From one memorable patient I learned just how separate emotional mood and physical mood can be. She related that she was vacuuming the living room carpet and suddenly became aware that she was wet. She realized that the way she was holding the vacuum in her hand and moving it back and forth had caused her to fantasize that it was her husband's penis.

She thought, I'll give him a real treat when he gets home. She made preparations, first calling her neighbor and arranging for her to take her two children for dinner and the evening. She fixed an appetizer and chilled a bottle of wine, bathed, perfumed, and put on a sexy outfit. Finally, she heard the car in the driveway. Then she heard the car door slam. Next, she heard her husband kick the kid's trike off the porch and curse as he slammed the door. He yelled at her about the trike as he came in. They had a loud, angry argument. She totally lost her mood. She changed her clothes and left the appetizer and wine in the fridge. The evening was quiet and tense, and they avoided each other.

Then, she said, when they were in bed, "Guess what he wanted to do? He wanted to have sex! I really told him off about treating me like that and then expecting sex. Then I pulled up my nightie, spread my legs, and said, 'Go ahead and do it and just see how much you enjoy it.' I was determined to punish him and give him the coldest, deadest sex imaginable. Can you believe that he did it! Almost immediately, I had a really strong orgasm. I didn't want to have it. I tried to stop it. I tried not to move but parts of me moved anyway. The strange thing was it felt really good, but I didn't enjoy it at all and was really mad when he finished."

"That's an amazing story, but I hope you two are getting along," I said.

She laughed and said, "Oh, we're fine. He held me for a while and then apologized profusely and told me what a terrible day he had at work. Then he told me how much he needed me and how much he loved me. We had a long talk. After a while we made love. No orgasm, but I really enjoyed it and went to sleep happy and satisfied."

This information helped me respond to a patient or two who told me they couldn't enjoy intercourse without having an orgasm.

"Really," I said. "Suppose your husband couldn't sleep and was tossing and turning because he had gotten some really bad news about his job or maybe one of his relatives, and you moved over to comfort him and hold him. You are trying to just console him. Then suppose you noticed that he was getting aroused, so you made love to him. Would you have had an orgasm?"

"I wouldn't have even thought about it," was the answer. "That wouldn't have been why I did it."

Other strange orgasm stories are brought to mind. Several patients told me that they had spontaneous orgasms as a result of intensely stressful or exciting situations. One that I remember was a college student about to take a big exam. She was very keyed up and anxious about it. As the professor came down the row handing out the exam, she was trembling. When he handed it to her, she had an orgasm. She was very embarrassed and looked around to see if anyone had noticed but, of course, no one was looking at her.

Interesting stuff, this physical versus emotional mood business. You ladies will want to remember that while women start off all emotional and become more and more physical as the affair matures; men start off all physical and get more emotional. I believe that men who love their spouses develop, over time, the ability to enjoy intercourse and be completely satisfied without having an orgasm. I think it's after age fifty or maybe sixty that this occurs. And, of course, the first time it happens, the woman is apt to ask, "Honey, are you all right? Did you come?" As they say, "What goes around comes around." Ladies, don't ask that! Just say something like "I hope that was as good for you as it was to me." You will likely get a very satisfied and satisfying response.

Nursing mothers have special problems with sex. I was once asked to give a talk about this to a La Leche League chapter. La Leche League is an organization that promotes breast feeding and provides education about it. I titled the talk, "Sex and the Nursing Mother." About twenty-five women, most with babies, some nursing, attended, along with a few husbands. I started by saying that most new mothers are educated a bit about this by their readings or by their obstetrician or nurse, and they learn that nursing suppresses the mother's estrogen level, causing their vagina to be dry, and that a lubricant is required for comfortable intercourse.

"Nowhere have I seen it written that nursing mothers suffer an almost complete loss of physical sex drive," I continued, and the room erupted! Every woman was talking to her neighbor or to her husband. It went on for perhaps a minute or two while I stood silent. When they quieted I said, "My, that certainly gave rise to some conversation."

"I think, Doctor," said a lady in the third row, "we were all saying to each other, 'Oh, thank goodness, I thought it was just me.'"

This was the fastest I ever hit pay dirt, that is, accomplished my goal to convince troubled women that they are normal. It also emphatically verified what I had been hearing from my patients. I had not learned about this in medical school or residency or read it anywhere, but I had heard it from so many patients I accepted it as fact. I recently went to the La Leche League website and noted that it lists eighty-three topics about breastfeeding but not one about sex and the nursing mother.

I told the group about comments that my patients had made. One said, "When the baby was a few weeks old, I became aware that I really wanted my husband to want me, but I didn't want to do anything about it." Another said, "I think nursing satisfies my need for physical closeness." The audience seemed to identify with these sentiments. Then I told them about the discussion I had with one patient about the "let down" reflex.

They, of course, were all aware that when they started to nurse the baby had to suck hard for some seconds before their milk lets down. I explained that the nipple stimulation causes a release of the hormone oxytocin from the pituitary gland that circulates in their bloodstream, causing the muscle cells around their milk ducts to contract. I mentioned that the same hormone release, caused by clitoral and vaginal stimulation during intercourse, played a part in a woman's orgasm and, many believe, caused the uterus to contract. Women are aware of their letdown reflex during the first week or so of nursing, because they can feel the uterine contraction and the lochia (old blood) that is expelled. Some women notice the similarity to orgasm and note a mild orgasm-like feeling when their milk lets down. I noticed a few heads nodding in the audience.

When I explained this to one patient, she said, "Oh, I'm so glad you told me because I had been thinking, Jane, you're not supposed to be feeling this way." And later on, after the baby starts to be fed food other than breast milk and mother's physical mood returns, orgasm will cause milk to squirt from both nipples.

What marvelous economy of design for the same physiologic mechanism that encourages women to have intercourse and get pregnant to also function to nourish the baby. A grand design indeed! Is it any wonder that a woman might not have the physical desire for intercourse while lactating. After all, she is having an orgasm-like experience five or six times a day.

The solution to the problem is simple. A woman simply needs to go back to the basics and recall that she first enjoyed intercourse emotionally and that the emotional satisfaction remained most important, even after she discovered her physical needs and abilities. She should satisfy her man quickly and well, perhaps surreptitiously applying a little lubricant first, then initiating the lovemaking, stimulating his brain with physical language and then expressing her satisfaction.

CHAPTER TEN

Advice For Young Women: The Formula For Sexcess

Unless a young woman finds her first love in a rational way and for the right reasons, I believe that it is very important that she get over that one. She can almost always do better. Most women find their first love after a date or when a previous acquaintance becomes a steady boyfriend. If sexual relations occur, it has different effects on each. Most young women seem to "fall in love" at this point and unconsciously become a little possessive, feeling that "now he is mine." Perceiving this, the young man often pushes back a little, doing things that express his independence. This is anxiety-producing for the woman, and she often prolongs the relationship by becoming compliant and striving to please. It is difficult to bring up the subject of marriage in this situation. If he then ends the relationship, she is devastated, especially if it has gone on for a while. She then suffers much and for a long time. I saw many young women in this state. Sadly, too many of them have this happen to them over and over.

After assuring these young women that they will look back upon this as a fortuitous event—and that they can undoubtedly do much better—I gave them my formula for success. I told them to regard every eligible man they encountered as a possible marriage partner and to evaluate him rationally before they became physically involved. "This is serious business," I said. They should develop a mental check list of attributes important to them, as well as the characteristics that immediately reject him.

"Grade him with your head before you get your bod involved," I would say. For instance, is he smart enough, kind enough, ambitious, caring, gentle, patient? Does he have some realistic idea of his future? As you get to know him, vet him out with friends and maybe on web sites that list sexual predators and arrest records. Make sure he is not a liar. If he thinks it's cute to fool or mislead people, lose him. He might make a great salesman, but he will be lying to you in no time. Watch out for addictive personalities—smoking, drinking, drugs, for instance. If a small amount of alcohol really effects him, it's a bad sign.

So if you decide that he is not marriage material but lots of fun—a hunk that lights your fire and you can handle it—take the proper precautions and have sex with him all you want. Just don't change your mind because he is good in bed. That's not going to eliminate his deficiencies. On the other hand, if you decide that he could be marriage material and you feel yourself getting emotionally involved, then, whatever you do, don't have sex with him. You can let him know that you want to—tease him a little—very little, then call a halt to the lovemaking by saying, "I'm just not ready yet." And stick to it!

If he asks if you are a virgin, act indignant and tell him, "That's for me to know and you to try to find out." One of two things will happen. He may stop calling and that will hurt because you are already emotionally involved. It won't hurt nearly as much, however, as it would if you have become intimate with him. You'll know what he was after, and that's a good reason for rejection. Or, he may start talking about a future with you! If that progresses well, then you can "be ready" when you want to, but now you will be able to talk about your future without making him feel possessed. God gave men a strong physical sex drive for a reason. It's to make him do brave things like making commitments and keeping them. You should brazenly exploit that!

This will seem very old-fashioned to many modern young women who hop in and out of bed with multiple men. Behaving in that way is self-destructive and it will be very difficult for them to find a good man with whom they can share a life. What you have is very precious and you are a fool to give it away indiscriminately. Relieving men of their sexual tension allows them to exploit you and never requires them to make a commitment.

Proper precautions include birth control and protection against disease. Far and away the best contraception is the oral contraceptives. They, however, do nothing to prevent disease.

Best not to tell him that you are on them, so that you can insist on him using a condom every time. Continue this until you know him well enough to believe that he was not promiscuous previously and is being monogamous with you. Then eliminating the condom might be an acceptable risk.

Watch out for the undersexed male. They are out there and you don't want one. I have had as patients several women, both married and unmarried, who have been involved with one. They can sweep a woman off her feet because they are low on the aggression scale, often gentle and caring. I asked one unmarried patient how often she was having sex and she said, "Oh, about once a week." Alarm bells went off in my head. I asked, "How often could you have sex, that is, how often do you have the opportunity?"

"Every day," she responded, "but that's what I like about him. He is not pushy and is very intellectual. We have long discussions and even read books together. He reads a chapter, then I read one. It's not just sex. I think I'll probably marry him."

"Fine," I said, "but I think you should find out if you can get him to have sex more than once a week. A woman must know that she can make her man want her whenever she wants to, and in my experience, if it's once a week before marriage, it's once a month after."

She returned a month later because of a recurrent vaginal infection and thanked me profusely. She reported that she had "dumped" him because she couldn't get him to make love more than once a week. She said that he always had some excuse, but once a week was his max. After the breakup, two of her friends told her, "Good, because he likes boys as much as he likes girls." I'm not saying that all undersexed males are gay. I think not, but I do know they are not good for women.

It's especially tragic if they marry, even more so if they have children. These men are usually good fathers, patient and gentle, doting on their kids. Interviewing a new patient, I would get her medical history, then ask my lead-in question: "Are you having any problems or difficulty with sex or intercourse?" There was a pause as I finished writing. I looked up and saw a tear running down her cheek. "I know that I'm not very attractive (she was gorgeous) but I always thought before marriage that we would make love more than once a month."

All I could tell her was that it wasn't her fault, and that her husband was distinctly abnormal and should see a doctor and have his hormones checked. Earlier, I had gotten one to go to a psychiatrist who helped him discover that he was gay, but this was obviously no help to the wife. These women are made to feel unattractive, and it's difficult for them to be convinced that they are not causing the problem. Once they became convinced, they quickly become dissatisfied with their situation and usually end up separating and eventually divorcing.

After listening to a few of these women and observing the outcome, I developed a hypothesis. All of the patients involved in this kind of situation were very attractive, and I questioned some about how they had settled on this particular man. One said that most of the men she dated were too aggressive, making a physical pass on the first or second date, which greatly upset her. If they called again, she refused to go out. Then she found one that wasn't that way. She felt that he really respected her and wasn't just after sex. He was very complimentary, often commenting on her clothes and hair style. So these women seemed to select this kind of man, perhaps because their upbringing had been strict and they were a little too scrupulous. I suggested that they be a little more gentle about fending off these aggressive males, that they might be rejecting some good men who are just a little overwhelmed.

Single girls who have become sexually active and are living at home with parents presented me with special problems, especially if they wanted me to keep this a secret. I certainly didn't want to rat them out and ruin the patient's trust in me. I did, however, want to get them on the pill. I always tried my best to talk to the mother and daughter separately.

Often, the mother had brought the daughter in because of some problem with her period or perhaps a vaginal discharge. Anything would do, and I would tell the young patient that I wanted her on the contraceptive pill for that reason, and I wanted her mother to know so the daughter didn't have to hide the pills, and so her parents would pay for them.

Many of these young patients would say, "She will ask you if I'm having sex." I assured them that only once did that happen, and my response was, "You're asking me if your daughter is having sex. I can't tell you that. She is your daughter. Why don't you ask her?"

Almost every one these mothers, when told that I wanted to put their daughter on the pill for this or that reason, would breathe a big sigh of relief and say, "That's fine, Doctor, I'm glad you told me."

I am sure that most of these women brought their daughters in because they feared they were having sex but didn't want to say it. It was, for me, a little sin of omission but one necessary to prevent unwanted pregnancies.

On occasion, I would see a young patient who had a valid medical reason to be put on oral contraceptives, but she would object, saying, "Doctor, I'm trying not to have sex with my boyfriend (or fiancée), and if you put me on the pill, I won't be able to hold off."

My response was, "Just because you're on the pill doesn't mean that you have to have sex; it just means you can if you want to. We have learned over and over that fear of pregnancy is not effective in preventing it. Now you can rationally decide. Do you really not want to have sex?" I recall a few patients that backed off on the physical aspect of their relationship and remained celibate until marriage.

A long-time patient called me one day and told me that she was bringing her sixteen-year-old daughter in because she had discovered that her daughter was sexually active. She wanted me to put her on the pill. I asked her, "How am I supposed to play this? Does your daughter know that you know?"

"Oh, she knows that I know," she said, "In fact, let me tell you what happened. My husband and I returned home last evening earlier than expected. He dropped me off at the door and drove the car around to the garage. I let myself in and walked into the living room and found my daughter and her boyfriend in the act."

I expressed my sympathy. She said, "But that's not the worst. Boyfriend jumped up, grabbed his underpants, and leaped through the nearest door, which put him in the headlights of my husband's car as he was pulling into the garage."

"What a shock that had to be," I said.

"At least they were practicing safe sex," she continued. "We both can attest to that."

CHAPTER ELEVEN

Circumcision Stories:
Do You Mind If I Cut In?

There is controversy about circumcisions to the point that there is even an organization dedicated to extirpate them entirely. They have a newsletter called "The NoCirc News," where grisly pictures of botched circumcisions are displayed. I'm not that sure if it's good or bad, and generally, after a little counseling, I left the decision up to the parents.

A majority of pediatricians at one time were against it, reporting that there was no valid medical reason for circumcision. The frequency of the operation then dropped off, and this resulted in more urinary tract infections in babies and young boys, which, before then, was very rare. Cancer of the penis, foreskin infections, and transmission of STDs is more common with the uncircumcised but still relatively rare. To address this, little boys—who frequently can't seem to remember to wash their elbows—were supposed to be taught from the earliest age to pull back the foreskin and wash under it when bathing.

My practice was in an area where the vast majority of boys were circumcised. I would ask the new parents to consider that their uncircumcised boy would be different from his peers. I allowed that this shouldn't be a problem if his daddy was uncircumcised. Most parents decided to have it done.

Pain was sometimes brought up as an issue, but this is almost entirely preventable with a penile nerve block. Now a few pointers for the ob resident: the sensory nerves come into the penis at ten and two o'clock, adjacent to the tiny veins. Each nerve sends a posterior branch to innervate the underside of the penis. These emanate from the main nerve about a centimeter above the juncture of the penis and abdominal wall. A little local anesthetic at ten and two, with a tiny 27-gauge, five-eighths-inch needle, then directing the needle upward for its full length to get each posterior branch, numbs the entire penis. It's so easy. It's not rocket science. It is important to wait four or five minutes for the drug to work before starting the procedure. This was my routine, and it was so effective that I always invited the mother and father to watch. I would tell them circumcision jokes while I had them captive. "There is a man who comes by the nursery every day to collect the foreskins. He tans them and sews them into little coin purses. He sells them for a lot of money because you rub them a little and they expand into a two-suiter," was one of my stories.

I had a lot of trouble getting my residents to use anesthesia for circumcisions because it takes a little longer, particularly the female residents. I required each resident to do five circumcisions under local anesthetic to demonstrate their proficiency and learn for themselves how peaceful it was, in contrast to having the baby screaming the whole time. I was appalled a few years later when I heard one of my female graduates tell a patient that anesthesia wasn't necessary because baby's nerves are not fully developed and they don't feel any pain during the procedure.

My chief resident, Duke, one year ahead of me in the program, was an excellent obstetrician/gynecologist. Duke was a large, jolly fellow universally liked by all. He was a master of self-deprecating humor and expressed one lament, which was, he claimed, the small size of his organ. He described himself as two hundred pounds of dynamite with a half-inch fuse. We got along famously, trusting each other implicitly, and working together on many cases.

One of these was a clinic (residents') patient who was admitted in labor with twins. I gave the anesthetic, a continuous epidural, while Duke did the delivery. She delivered twin boys. The next day I saw her on rounds, and she told me that she was so happy with her care that she named her boys after us—Eban and Duke. I thanked her and went to the nursery to circumcise the boys. The mother declined to watch. The babies were placed side by side on the nursery counter, and when their diapers were removed I was amazed at the difference in them. They were obviously not identical twins. Twin A had a very large penis while twin B's was tiny. Out I went to talk with the mother. "Which twin is which?" I asked her. By the grace of God, it came out right. Twin B was Duke.

As I trimmed the boys, I asked the nurse to put out a stat page for Duke. When he came in the door, I covered the sites with towels, told him the story, and asked him if he could tell which was which. As I pulled the towels off he looked from one to the other. His hands flew to his face as he wailed, "Oh no!"

Yes, we did have our fun.

CHAPTER TWELVE

Endometriosis: The Mystery and What You Should Know About It

Endometriosis is a disease poorly understood by most women, and its treatment has not improved for several decades. Still of unproven cause, it is associated with infertility and seems to afflict women who delay child-bearing. It disproportionately occurs in Caucasian and Oriental women, and it is rare in African-American women.

Hormonally sensitive cells like those that line the uterine cavity develop in or are deposited on pelvic and/or abdominal organs. These cells, like the cells in the uterus, respond to monthly hormonal changes, in effect, degenerating at the end of the cycle into menstrual discharge. The ones in the uterus can, of course, drain out through the cervix and vagina, but the cells on the surface of the uterus, tubes, ovaries, bowel and pelvic walls, etc., have nowhere to go. They form blood blister-like deposits that are sticky and cause tenderness and pain at period time for most affected women. Over time, these can enlarge and form cystic deposits full of chocolate-like fluid (chocolate cysts). They also cause dense scaring, resulting in attachment to the peritoneum (lining layer) of the pelvic and abdominal cavities and adjacent organs, such as ovaries and bowel.

To be cured requires that these patients wait for menopause to occur when the disease becomes inactive or undergo a complete hysterectomy, including the ovaries. Pregnancy, if it occurs, seems to put the disease into remission for varying periods of time. Hormonal treatment, as with combination oral contraceptives, do help some patients, but many women have side effects. Young women who are affected, especially those who might desire more children, should procrastinate as long as they can stand it, as they try to get pregnant, or wait for menopause. A small percentage of patients have little discomfort with the disease and may be unaware that they have it. In them, it can progress to the point that they are found at checkup to have large, firm pelvic masses—a frozen pelvis, in gyn terminology—difficult to distinguish from ovarian cancer.

When I was chief resident, I scrubbed on a private case with a gynecologist who seldom got a chief resident to assist him because he never let the resident do anything other than hold retractors and observe. Dr. Grad was a distinguished gynecologist and an excellent and precise but slow surgeon usually assigned a first- or second-year resident who could profit a lot by watching his precise technique. I noted nothing challenging on the surgery schedule the following day, and because I liked and respected Dr. Grad so much, decided to assist him one more time. I did so even though I knew that I could do the case in two hours, while I would probably spend three hours or more with him.

I worked up his patient, who was admitted the night before surgery, with a diagnosis of advanced ovarian cancer. On the pelvic exam she had the typical frozen pelvis, a large, solid, fixed mass extending almost to the umbilicus. It felt like cancer to me until I searched out the uterus, which can sometimes be identified at the bottom of the mass. It was pushed forward under the bladder. Carefully feeling the anterior wall of the uterus through the vaginal wall, I felt hard little masses, like BB shot. Only endometriosis can feel like that. My diagnosis was severe endometriosis.

Scrubbing at the sink the next morning, Dr. Grad, having read my admission history and physical, said to me, "So, Dr. Rock, you think Mrs. Smith has endometriosis?"

"No, Dr. Grad," I said, "I know she has endometriosis."

He chuckled and said, "Well, for her sake, I certainly hope you're right, but that's ovarian cancer or I've never felt it before."

Dr. Grad was trained by general surgeons at the university hospital, which mostly cared for African-American patients and had likely seldom seen endometriosis there. I watched him make the abdominal incision, and as he opened the peritoneum the chocolate-like fluid ran out.

"Well, I will be," he said as he paused with the skin knife in his hand.

The scrub nurse, clean knife in hand, impatiently asked, "Knife, Dr. Grad?"

"Give it to Dr. Rock," he said. "He made the diagnoses, so he can take it out."

That was a proud moment for me! I was a little disappointed that he never asked me how I knew. Now, years later, CAT scans or an MRI can likely differentiate between endometriosis and ovarian cancer. I preferred making the diagnosis in the office and saving the patient worry, expense, and X-ray exposure.

While stationed at Rader Army Clinic, a patient was referred by a general medical officer for presumed ovarian cancer when I again diagnosed endometriosis. She did not believe me as I referred her in late October to Bethesda Navel Hospital for surgery. I told her that I would call her on Thanksgiving to wish her a happy one. I did, and she reported that I was right.

Endometriosis patients that come to hysterectomy are extremely grateful women and have a wonderful post-operative course. They had usually suffered much for a long time and when the surgery was over the post-operative pain was often less than what they were putting up with, and it lessened every day. Their husbands were happy as well.

We had just moved into a new neighborhood and made friends with Jake and Adel and their two teenaged daughters. We, with our teenagers, went with them and several other neighbors to a southern lake for a vacation. I noticed that Adel was suffering and inquired as to what was wrong. She said that she had very painful periods and constant pelvic tenderness. Her family doctor was not helping her much. After hearing this and taking a little more history, I said, "Adel, I know what is wrong with you."

She made an appointment with me and soon had her hysterectomy. She did extremely well, and she and Jake were very grateful. She had been so tender that they had been unable to have sex for some time. A couple of months later, at dinner, Jake asked me what my usual hysterectomy fee was. He was dismayed at the small amount insurance had paid and wanted to pay me the difference.

"Don't worry about it, Jake," I said. "Just pay me what it was worth to you."

Without hesitation he exclaimed, "Oh, Eban, I could never afford that!"

CHAPTER THIRTEEN

Ultrasound: Believing is Not Always Seeing

Being in on the early use of ultrasound provided me with a better perspective than many of my colleagues. This helped me avoid pitfalls in a number of areas. One was in the diagnosis of placenta previa.

The placenta (afterbirth) normally implants high in the uterus but occasionally it implants low, sometimes even over the cervix. This is known as placenta previa (afterbirth coming first). As the cervix begins to thin and dilate during the last half of pregnancy, the lower part of the placenta tears loose from its attachment to the uterus, causing bleeding. Complete placenta previa covers the entire cervical opening and necessitates a caesarian section. The placenta is easily visualized by ultrasound and the report might be: either partial or complete placenta previa. Terri's case illustrates the usual course of the condition but not the usual treatment.

At about twenty-eight weeks gestation, Terri called me because of heavy vaginal bleeding. After hospital admission the bleeding stopped. The sonogram (ultrasound) report read "complete placenta previa." Two units of compatible blood were prepared and held because Terri's blood count remained acceptable. The active fetus was determined to be in good condition. The bleeding soon stopped, as it usually does. The following day Terri was sent home under very reduced activity, and a short series of steroid injections was started—I made home visits—to hasten fetal lung maturity. Expectant management is in order for this condition. Bleeding will recur off and on but almost always stops in a reasonable period of time. Of course, each episode requires readmission and evaluation until fetal maturity is assured, at which time the caesarian section is done.

Terri had two additional admissions before the final one, which came at almost thirty-six weeks gestation. Bleeding moderately at arrival, she was taken directly to the operating room where a general anesthetic was administered and all preparations for caesarian section were completed. Not being a total believer of the shadows and echoes of a sonogram providing an accurate diagnosis of complete placenta previa, however, I decided to do a double-setup exam. With prepping and draping for the operation accomplished, I did a very gentle vaginal exam (traditionally a no-no, for fear of increasing the bleeding).

With my gloved fingertip I felt the gritty surface of the placenta covering a third of the five-centimeter dilated cervix, so it was not a complete placenta previa. The rest of the cervical opening revealed the smooth membrane of the amniotic sac. The fetal head was a centimeter or so above and not yet engaged in the pelvis. I decided to rupture the membranes (another no-no, for fear of a prolapsed umbilical cord), knowing that I could deliver the baby by caesarian in a minute or two if things went awry.

I made a small hole in the membranes and slowly leaked the fluid, causing the baby's head to settle into the pelvis. A spontaneous uterine contraction pushed it firmly against the cervix, compressing the bleeding cervix beneath the detached portion of the placenta and completely stopping the bleeding. I attached the fetal monitor electrode and verified that the fetus was in excellent condition.

The general anesthetic was discontinued and Terri woke up. Labor was augmented with oxytocin and an epidural was administered. In about two hours, Terri had a normal delivery of a healthy baby boy. Terri, her husband, and I were delighted that she avoided a caesarean section. I'm sure that some of my colleagues would have faulted this management as risky, especially those who had more than a 30 percent caesarian section rate.

Diagnosing the sex of a fetus should be a slam-dunk with the modern, high definition ultrasound machines, but it was not always so. One of my chief residents, Dr. Kaplan, scanned his wife to discover the sex of their baby and saw, he thought, boy parts, only to be embarrassed when she delivered a girl some weeks later. This illustrates just one of the many reasons that a doctor should not take care of his family and relatives. I had a lot of fun with this a few days later.

The director of the department, Dr. Zee, took a weekend off to go out of town, and I covered his practice. His patient, Mrs. Whitt, who was scheduled to have a repeat caesarian on Monday, called me in the wee hours of Saturday morning and reported that her water had broken. She was not in labor and wanted to wait for Dr. Zee on Monday. She wanted no part of me.

I gently explained that it would be too dangerous for her to wait; that she would probably start labor and have to rush to the hospital, or if she didn't do that, she had an increasing risk of infection, or having a number of other bad things happen. I pleaded with her to come in and have her baby and she reluctantly agreed. This was her fourth caesarian section. Their three children were girls. As my assistant, Dr. Kaplan, and I draped her for surgery, Mrs. Whitt was obviously in a snit. She wouldn't even look at me.

I tried to lighten her up by saying, "Maybe this one will be a boy."

"Ultrasound said it's another girl," she snapped and turned her head away.

A few minutes later I took great delight in holding the baby's bottom above the ether screen drape and showing her and her husband their baby's boy parts. I never saw a woman cheer up so fast.

Then that light bulb lurking invisibly over my head flashed on. The realization that the Kaplans and the Whitts had a similar problem suddenly occurred to me. I reintroduced Mr. and Mrs. Whitt to Dr. Kaplan. I explained that the Kaplans had lots of boy baby clothes at home that they didn't need, and I surmised that the Whitts had lots of girl baby clothes that they wouldn't need, and I proceeded to try to broker a clothes exchange as we finished the operation.

What fun, indeed. Later Mrs. Whitt wrote me the nicest note saying that she had checked me out with friends and discovered that she couldn't have been in better hands—except for Dr. Zee's, of course.

CHAPTER FOURTEEN

Incompetent Cervix: A Rare and Misdiagnosed Event

Another area where ultrasound cannot provide an accurate diagnosis, in my opinion, is in the diagnosis of incompetent cervix. This is a very rare condition almost always occurring during the first pregnancy, caused by a very weak or pliable cervix not rigid enough to hold a pregnancy long enough for the fetus to be viable. The fetus is usually lost at about twenty weeks of gestation. I believe that this is often misdiagnosed, leading to unnecessary and often ineffective treatment.

The patient usually comes to the doctor complaining of a bulge at the vaginal opening, which is the bag of waters that has hour-glassed through the cervix and passively dilated it without perceptible contractions. Sometimes she has leaking fluid because the bag of waters has broken. In both cases, if asked, the patient will report that she felt a sensation of vaginal or rectal fullness or pressure for a day or more before the bulge or leakage of water occurred. This, I believe, is caused by the leading point of the bag of waters, which has come through the cervix and into the vagina.

This critical history is absent in cases of premature labor, which is sometimes misdiagnosed as incompetent cervix, especially by doctors who think surgery first. I do not believe that true incompetent cervix can be diagnosed by ultrasound before the pregnancy is lost. It's very important to make an accurate diagnosis, because the treatment of incompetent cervix starts the patient on a slippery slope if she wants more children, leading to multiple additional operations.

The treatment for incompetent cervix is the surgical closure of the cervix, best done with a circular ribbon or band of surgical fabric in an operation called "cervical cerclage." A less effective method, in my view, is to suture the cervix closed with strong suture material. Progesterone suppositories, used to treat premature labor, may be helpful but probably will not suffice for true cervical incompetence. The vaginal approach for the operation is the best, and it is a relatively minor operation for the patient. When the time comes for delivery, hopefully near term, the fabric or suture can be removed and the patient allowed to labor.

About half of the time, the cervix immediately dilates several centimeters when the cerclage is removed, and labor progresses normally. In some, the cervix will only dilate partially, presumably because of scarring of the cervix from the operation, and a caesarian section is needed. If another pregnancy occurs, the cerclage operation needs to be repeated.

Sometimes, the fabric band is completely healed over and can be left in and the baby delivered by caesarian section. This avoids another cerclage operation with the next pregnancy. However, her chance of getting pregnant with the cerclage in place is much reduced until it is removed. When pregnancy occurs, back in goes the cerclage.

A case history illustrates why I don't think incompetent cervix can be diagnosed by ultrasound prior to a pregnancy loss. I noticed one day that a cervical cerclage operation was scheduled on a hospital clinic patient (a resident's patient) and asked the chief resident the details. She said that the perinatologist (maternal-fetal medicine specialist) had diagnosed it by ultrasound and ordered the operation.

Being ultimately responsible for the clinic patients, I inquired of the perinatologist how he made the diagnosis. He told me that this was the patient's first pregnancy, and she was about twenty-five weeks into gestation, and he had verified by sonogram that the cervix was incompetent. I asked him to bring the patient back and show me. The cervix was definitely thinned out, and when the perinatologist pressed on the maternal abdomen to put pressure on the uterus, the bag of waters appeared to open the cervix perhaps two or three centimeters and actually bulge a bit through the cervical opening—a very impressive sight, indeed. Nevertheless, knowing how rare the condition is and knowing of no convincing evidence that it could be diagnosed in this manner, I demurred.

With both parents in the ultrasound room, I discussed the diagnosis. I pointed out that incompetent cervix is quite rare, and that this method to diagnose it is unproven. I also informed them that the treatment has consequences for subsequent pregnancies, which would require additional surgery. I said that, at this point, only God could know if she has an incompetent cervix, and I left it up to them to decide if they wanted the operation. They decided not to have it. She went home on restricted activities, especially no sexual intercourse, until thirty-five weeks of gestation.

Two weeks before her due date, at thirty-eight weeks, the patient came in with false labor. After verifying that the fetus was in good condition, she was sent home. She returned at term, in good labor, and a short time later delivered a seven-pound baby. Incompetent cervix? Definitely not!

Other unindicated surgeries occur under the title of "Plastic Surgery." In the dressing booth in each of my exam rooms, a sign was posted: If you are thinking of having any plastic surgery, please discuss it with Dr. Rock. Cosmetic plastic surgery is different from reconstructive plastic surgery, the former being entirely elective surgery, usually based on a person's perception of some inadequacy or defect in appearance. Reconstructive plastic surgery addresses real defects such as cleft lips, birth defects, deforming injuries, burns, etc.

Cosmetic plastic surgery is overdone, in my opinion, and I did my best to talk patients out of it. My motivation was increased if the patient was in her late thirties or forties. What most of these ladies needed, in my opinion, was counseling for their midlife crisis.

Breast augmentation is especially overdone, both in frequency and implant size. Women need to know how men really feel about women's breasts. It's simple: they just like them, and if a woman acts like she knows that her breasts are attractive to her man, they will be. I told my patients that if they have their breasts enlarged, they run the risk of going from attractive to gaudy, or even garish. And there are definite downsides to this type of surgery.

A big downside is cost. The procedures are not covered by insurance, and practitioners charge what the public will bear and usually want the payment up front. Doctors with income as their prime motivation are attracted to specialties like this. There are male chauvinist pigs among them who routinely stuff in the biggest implants possible. These stretch the overlying breast tightly, which could reduce the blood supply to the covering tissue and may contribute to fibrosis, causing hardening.

Implants can leak, and many do after several years. Silicone-filled implants have a more natural feel, but when they leak, cause hardening. The many diseases blamed on silicone are no longer thought to be from this inert substance. This after many lawyers garnered massive disability awards for clients and huge incomes for themselves. Saline-filled implants can and do leak, causing flattening and a crinkly sound when the thick plastic bag is pressed on, such as during an embrace.

A patient called me about fifteen years after she acquired saline-filled implants and reported that one had gone flat. A few months later, the other one went. She put up with this for a while but couldn't tolerate the lumpiness and crinkling and eventually went back to the plastic surgeon. She refused new implants. It cost her many thousands of dollars to have the plastic removed and her "puppy dog ears," as she called them, reduced and made perkier.

I have to confess that I was not very effective at talking patients out of the procedure but was much better at dissuading them from having too large an implant placed. I also admit that until they started to have problems, they really liked the results.

I once gave an epidural for the labor and delivery of an anesthesiologist's wife. This was at the time when my group and I were the only source for this in the city. It went well, and at the six-week checkup, she brought me a bottle of Chateau Lafite Rothschild 1966.

Years later, in my second career, I told this story to my colleague who was a retired plastic surgeon and serious wine buff.

"Eban," he said, "that's amazing. I did a breast augmentation on a colleague's wife and they gave me a case of Chateau Lafite Rothschild 1976."

Shows how an epidural stacks up against a good boob job!

CHAPTER FIFTEEN

Telephone Management: Where Talk is Cheap

How would I handle the telephone if I were in practice today? I can't even comprehend how well doctor-patient communication might—and does—function with cell phones, email, Facebook, Twitter, and blogs. An answering service would still be a necessity, I believe. I had a good one, and I made an effort to train every operator in how I wanted my calls handled. Unless they were calls that could obviously wait, that is, appointment calls, advertisements, surveys, and so forth, I wanted them relayed to me promptly. I made it a point to never yell at or even sound irritated if given a call that was obviously unnecessary. I called patients as soon as possible. This was not unduly burdensome because as a partner in a group, I was on call only every fourth day. When I accepted a position as residency program director at a large hospital, my major source of income was salary from the hospital. I had a small practice—in effect a concierge practice—so the calls were not burdensome.

Today, I think I would give trusted patients direct access by cell phone, texting, or email, as all are quicker and more reliable than calling them back. Those patients would have to have demonstrated over time that they were reasonable and considerate. There are many advantages to providing this level of service. It builds a great doctor-patient relationship, and knowing that the doctor is so readily available prevents patient anxiety. Proper questioning of the patient on the phone usually yields a diagnosis and saves the patient a trip to the emergency room. These days, many patients are sent there without any kind of screening (triage), resulting in patient inconvenience, ED overload, and much unnecessary cost.

If consideration of the patient's chief complaint and recent history doesn't make a diagnosis apparent, then a brief review of systems is in order. This only takes a minute or two and yields great benefits. For example, a patient called me because of right lower quadrant pain. Appendicitis? She had a normal appetite and no nausea, making that unlikely. Review of systems revealed that she was feeling chilly (fever?), had a bad cough that was productive, and she was a little short of breath. I suspected right lower lobe pneumonia, and that diagnosis was confirmed by chest x-ray.

Her pain was an example of "referred" pain, which is internal pain, misinterpreted to be in a different location, like for instance, cardiac pain to the left arm, gall bladder pain to the right shoulder, and so forth. This occurs because the body is not good at identifying the location of internal pain, confusing it with an area of the external body, the nerves of which enter the spinal cord next to the nerves from the internal site.

A huge benefit of doing a review of systems occurs when the review comes up completely negative. When this occurred, I would give the patient my impression and, always, a way out. I would say, "Nothing you are telling me rings any bells indicating a serious problem, but I'm not the one having the pain (discomfort, sensation, feeling, bleeding). But if you are concerned, I'll be glad to see you or have you seen in the emergency room."

It was incredible how the patients sorted themselves out. The vast majority would say something like, "Oh, no, Doctor, if you're not concerned, then I'm not, either. I'll take some aspirin and if it persists, I'll call the office tomorrow."

Occasionally a patient would say, "I really would feel better if I were seen," and I always found them to have a significant ailment.

The biggest benefit is that the patient knows you care. You demonstrated interest, let her share in the decision-making, and didn't blow her off (take two aspirin and call me in the morning). Treat patients in this way, and you will be trusted and liked. This is very gratifying work.

It is very important for a doctor not to sound irritated when talking to a patient, especially over the phone. It took me some time and a few mistakes to develop the self-discipline to control my tone of voice in the middle of the night when hearing a seemingly frivolous complaint about a problem that had been going on for five days. My previous mistakes were being short with patients, then later discovering they had a serious problem. When I found myself getting irritated, I forced myself to sound sweeter and sweeter, sometimes syrupy sweet. My wife would tell me that it drove her nuts to listen to me. To handle this internally, I would sometimes have to think, If the dumb bunny falls for this line, she really is stupid.

My senior partner taught me a wonderful office routine. If a patient was seen or talked to on the phone and perhaps a prescription given, a callback routine was used. Under the desk in our work center was a vertical arrangement of five boxes labeled Monday through Friday. Let's say a patient was seen on Monday and acute cystitis (bladder infection) was diagnosed and a prescription given. The doctor might write, "Call Wednesday" at the end of his note. The head nurse, who checked every chart, would then put the chart in the Wednesday box. Sometime during that day, the nurse would anticipate the doctor coming out of an exam room, and she would call the patient and park her on hold until the doctor could pick up the call.

The doctor would find the chart on the counter in front of his phone, open to his Monday note, which might have a red eight written on it, indicating the phone line where the patient was waiting.

"Mrs. Smith, Dr. Rock. How are you feeling? Is the medicine working?" These were generally short conversations and usually very gratifying. It is always nice to know that you cured someone. This had many positive aspects. Usually, when you called, the patient, sounding surprised, would say something like "I'm feeling much better, Doctor. Thank you."

Often the patient was so shocked at getting the call that she would have no additional questions. Sometimes you would discover that the patient, who appeared to be dying on Monday, hadn't even filled the prescription (20 percent or more) and that could be discussed. You would occasionally discover allergic reactions to your medicine. The patients loved the care. It was a practice-builder. Patients sent their friends and relatives, and all of it was gratifying for the doctor.

All those are good reasons to check on patients, but the real important one is that sometimes the patients are not better. Sometimes they are worse. Sometimes they have developed localizing signs telling you that you missed the diagnoses of a serious problem. Who better to find this than you, instead of a doc-in-a-box—urgent care center doctor— who, with the diagnosis now obvious might ask, "Your doctor said you had WHAT?" The patient might have gone there because she is upset because of the money she spent for your office visit and more money for the prescription, which isn't working. It is gratifying to find your mistakes before the patient has much trouble and gets angry.

Sometimes a phone call to a patient pays off big time. One day, for some reason, I found myself thinking of a patient of whom I was especially fond of and had not seen for some time. At her last checkup well over a year before, we had a somewhat sensitive conversation, and I worried that because of that she felt too uncomfortable to return. I fretted about that for a week or two and finally called her. I told her that I missed her and realized that perhaps she didn't want to see me again and wanted to be sure she was getting her checkups. She assured me that she would never see anyone else and had just been too busy but would call and make an appointment. I did not recall that at her last visit I had noted that she was quite a bit overdue for her mammogram, and I had chided her about that. She remembered that, however, and scheduled one before she came in. Guess what? That mammogram discovered an early breast cancer. It was very early and the surgeon's recommendation was to have a lumpectomy, and I concurred. She opted for a mastectomy and is fine and with no recurrence years later. She credits me with saving her life. I thank my Lord for nudging me to call her.

The key to making telephone checks work was to have a system. The nurse did the work by calling the patient. She got the busy signals, wrong numbers, ten-ring no answers, and waits to get mommy on the phone. The doctor doesn't have time for this. Senior partner's mantra was, "Don't be penny wise and pound foolish. Hire enough good people to do everything they can do for you so that you can spend all of your time being with or talking to the patients."

Another positive effect of telephone follow-up, I believe, is that it prevents lawsuits. All of us make mistakes and/or miss things. I did at least once, and this is how I found out about it. I was finishing up a routine checkup when the patient said to me, "You know, Doctor, my sister is so-and so."

Oh no, I thought to myself. Not her. I screwed up her case. I caused her a lot of trouble.

"And you know, Doctor," the patient went on to say, "the family wanted her to sue you. My sister said, 'Sue Dr. Rock? He's the best doctor I've ever had. I wouldn't even think about suing him.'"

I realized that my good rapport had saved me from a lawsuit. If you have given the patient good and compassionate care, and the patient perceived that you liked him or her, they will not want to sue you when something goes awry. Having suffered only one lawsuit in thirty-five years of practice, and that one frivolous, I rest my case.

Another example of how patient rapport heads off lawsuits involved an inadvertent, unwanted circumcision. During residency, one of the busiest doctors on our service, Dr. Fuzzy, felt that he was too busy to do circumcisions. He paid the ob chief resident $25 each to do them for him. This was not ghost surgery, as Dr. Fuzzy told the patient that his chief resident would do it. Junior residents couldn't wait to become chief residents and get to that franchise. Dr. Fuzzy delivered lots of babies.

Dr. Fuzzy also played a lot of golf. He frequently took long weekend trips to play the best courses. He brought in patients on Thursday for induction of labor and moved up scheduled caesarean sections a few days, so he didn't miss too many deliveries. One Saturday, the chief resident went to the nursery to see if there were any babies of Dr. Fuzzy's to circumcise. There were five. She did all five. One of them was not supposed to be circumcised and no permit had been signed. On Monday morning, the parents met with their attorney in the mother's hospital room and planned on suing the resident. The attorney didn't mention that in addition to the resident, the hospital and Dr. Fuzzy would have to be named.

I was in the nurses' station when Dr. Fuzzy arrived on Tuesday morning. I heard the head nurse tell him what had transpired. He cursed a blue streak. Embarrassed, I left and went to visit my patient, who was in a semi-private room, one patient to the right and one to the left as you entered the room. As I talked to my patient, Dr. Fuzzy breezed in behind me to see his patient.

I heard him ask how she was doing and if she felt ready to go home. Then he said, "Mrs. Jones, the reason Dr. Morse circumcised your boy is because I told her to. The reason I told her to was because he really needed it."

"Oh," said Mrs. Jones, "that's okay then. I'm so glad you told me."

End of lawsuit! Dr. Fuzzy handled it exactly right. He didn't blame anyone else and took full responsibility himself. He had the rapport, and he banked on it.

One of my chief residents, Dr. Stouffer, did a hysterectomy on a clinic patient and left a sponge (cloth lap tape) in the patient. This occurred after the sponge count was reported as correct when the peritoneum—the innermost layer of the abdominal wall—was about closed. The lead-marked sponges (identifiable on x-ray) were replaced on the Mayo instrument tray with lap tapes (two-by-four-inch rectangular cotton fabric) which lack the lead markings. The scrub nurse then turned her back to the operation to count instruments on the back table. Some bleeding welled up through the last inch or two of the peritoneal opening. The resident put in three lap tapes to pack back the intestines, identify the source, and suture it. He then removed only two.

The patient recovered uneventfully and went home in five days. After a week, she called with pain under her incision. The resident brought her in to check, and he and his supervising consultant noted that the incision appeared to be healing well. The patient had no fever and was up and about and functioning normally. Her only finding was tenderness under the incision. He discussed the possibility of adhesions between the layers of the abdomen, assured her that the transverse incision was very strong, and said she should stay active and the adhesions should stretch and become less painful. He called her a few days later and found that she was no better. Dr. Stouffer was one of my most personable and caring residents. He brought her back to the clinic, and he and his consultant examined her again. The decision was made to explore the incision, and the lap tape was found and removed.

After the surgery, a dejected Dr. Stouffer came to my office, gave me his report, and asked me what he should tell the patient.

"What do I tell you to tell patients?" I asked.

"Tell the truth," he said.

"Do so," I said, "and explain to her exactly how it happened. That's not too complicated for a lay person to understand. Specifically absolve the circulating nurse and scrub nurse of any blame, take full responsibility yourself, and express all the sorrow and remorse you can muster."

He must have done a good job because as he explained this to the patient and her husband in their hospital room, the patient was patting his hand and saying, "Don't worry, Dr. Stouffer. I'll do fine. You listened to me. You didn't let me linger. I'll do fine." She did very well, and there was no mention of legal action. Rapport is everything.

Had she taken this to an attorney, the hospital's defense attorney would have simply asked "How much does the patient want?" and a substantial settlement would have been negotiated. There is no defense for this kind of action. Res ipsa loquitur—the thing itself speaks—is the legal term to describe this kind of negligence.

CHAPTER SIXTEEN

Training Residents: The Short List of What They Must Know

Using good medical judgment is also a deterrent to lawsuits, but it is hard to teach. To begin with, common sense is required. Up-to-date knowledge of one's specialty is obviously necessary, as well as the knowledge of what you don't know and a willingness to admit it. It helps to be unencumbered by ego and to always put your patient first. Being ethical is critical.

Patients are often the last to know how good their doctor is. They can judge whether they get good service, and they readily perceive if their doctor cares for and likes them, but how good the doctor may actually be is hard for another doctor to know, let alone a lay person. Nurses are good at knowing, although some are unduly impressed by personality, looks, or bedside manner.

The best at knowing are residents training in a particular doctor's specialty. They see the doctor at his/her best and worst, rested and tired, relaxed and stressed, methodically working or rushed, and they have an extensive knowledge of the specialty themselves. Surgical doctors who do a lot of unindicated operations are often the best technicians, and I would go to one of those if I was positive that I needed the operation.

When I was chief resident, one of my very ethical teachers was lamenting to me that we, the residents, had too much exposure to a gynecologist, a superb technician, who did a lot of poorly-indicated cases and would be corrupted by him.

"Have no worries," I told him. "We learn technique from him, but we learn indications from you and teachers like you."

In my training, I observed fellow residents who themselves did not have good judgment recommend the same doctors that I would have. They recognized good judgment and skill even though they didn't have it themselves.

It is very easy to do unindicated hysterectomies. There are many women who, at various times in their lives, would love to get rid of their uterus. Bleeding occurs when it shouldn't; it cramps; it gets pregnant. There are many reasons women are happy to hear their doctor say, "You need a hysterectomy."

The problem is that they don't know enough about the risks and possible unintended consequences of that major surgical procedure to make a valid judgment. The ethical gynecologist many times can and should provide a solution to the patient's problem with a simpler, less risky treatment. If the patient still wants a hysterectomy, the ethical physician should try to talk the patient out of it. Of course, there are less ethical gynecologists who will gladly do it. The excuse they often give is that if they don't do it, someone else will. One can excuse a lot of sins with this kind of reasoning. It's important to know that if something goes wrong and the patient sues—and the only indication for surgery is that the patient wanted it—the doctor will lose.

Doctors who blow their own horn about how smart they are and how important they are often get an extensive following. In my training years, I often noted that patients seemed to rave most over the biggest quacks. If things went awry, these doctors were also more likely to get sued. If you had the patient believing that you were infallible, and things didn't go right, the patient was first shocked, then disappointed, then often became angry.

There are some things that definitely interfere with medical judgment. Being emotionally involved with a patient certainly can, which is why most doctors will not care for family members or close relatives. If it even occurs to a doctor how much money will be made doing a procedure, judgment will likely be flawed. Doctors need to insulate themselves from what their procedures pay by having a good business manager handle that part of the practice.

Training residents in a surgical specialty such as obstetrics and gynecology, as I did for twenty-five years, is very gratifying work. I enjoyed helping them learn and grow and develop the knowledge, judgment, and technical expertise needed so that by the time they graduated, they were comfortable with decision-making, delivering babies, and doing surgical procedures on their own. Ob/gyn requirements are for four years of training after graduation from medical school and that generally is after four years of pre-med in college. Sub-specialization as in gynecologic oncology, maternal fetal medicine, reproductive endocrinology, and urogynecology require an additional two to four years. Some of the other surgical residencies are much longer, perhaps eight years for neurosurgery.

For residents to gain the technical expertise needed, they must do a lot of surgery. Watching and assisting a skilled surgeon operate is valuable for residents in the early years of training, but they must eventually do it themselves—over and over again. This starts in medical school where students are taught sterile technique, knot-tying, and basic suturing. Suturing of lacerations in the emergency room is experienced by third-year students. They also begin to assist on major surgical cases, usually holding retractors. During the end of their third year, students apply to residency programs.

First-year ob/gyn residents deliver a lot of babies in most programs, but they are also involved in gynecologic surgery. Many residencies utilize animal labs and simulation experiences where residents develop the hand-eye coordination needed. This is especially true for laparoscopic surgery where realistic simulators allow the resident to look at a TV screen and manipulate viewed instruments to cut and suture inert materials and specimens.

In the operating room, they assist on major cases and do minor ones. By the second year, residents are doing some major cases, usually on resident clinic patients under the supervision of senior residents and faculty. While assisting staff physicians on private patients, they will begin to do less critical parts of the operation, again under direct supervision. Third- and fourth-year residents have increasing responsibility in managing high-risk obstetric patients, and those that have demonstrated competence may be doing entire major gynecologic operations, including those on many of the private patients of staff physicians. This may give non-medical people pause, but it is absolutely necessary to train the needed numbers of specialists, and it provides benefits to patients that only a teaching hospital can supply.

Teaching hospitals must stay on the cutting edge of medical expertise and provide up-to-date equipment and instruction for resident physicians. Accrediting agencies for the hospital and the residency programs regularly inspect and verify that their requirements are being met. Patients on the teaching services of these hospitals have the advantage of being cared for by several resident physicians, in addition to their private physician, and one or more of these residents are in-house twenty-four hours a day. In addition, ob/gyn residencies are required to have an in-house attending faculty physician provide consultation and supervision for these residents twenty-four hours a day, seven days a week.

Residents in the last year or two of their training program are generally very proficient technically. They are often doing eight to twelve major cases a week and their hands are lightning fast and accurate. They are, after all, at the peak of their physical being, usually in their early thirties. If they were athletes, they would be at the top of their game. They have enormous stamina, are highly motivated, and extremely interested in their work. The patient's private physician, who generally acts as the first assistant, watches every move and has vast experience in recognizing unusual or rare occurrences, such as variations in anatomy, sudden unanticipated events, or equipment problems. It has been said the hardest part of doing an operation is knowing what to do next, and that's what the experienced attending physician knows.

In my position I cared for many nurses and doctors who knew exactly how I delegated surgical cases. I often discussed this with them in the office pre-op visit. Most expressed opinions, as did an anesthesiologist who had staffed my surgical cases many times. Dr. Carlton, with her first pregnancy, required a caesarean section. In the labor room beforehand, I said, "Jane, you have seen me do many sections and know that if a qualified resident scrubs with me, he or she will do the procedure."

"Eban," she said, "your residents are really good, and you watch them like a hawk. Don't change a thing for me."

Occasionally, a patient that I scheduled for surgery would at the pre-op visit say to me, "You are going to actually do the surgery, are you not?" I explained to them that I was in the teaching business and if a qualified resident scrubbed with me, he or she would likely do much of it. After giving them the information above, I would say, "If I do the whole operation, you will be on the table under anesthesia a bit longer than if I supervise a resident who does it. I'm not doing ten or twelve surgeries a week as they are."

They all accepted this plan.

EPILOGUE

Obstetrics and gynecology and anesthesiology, as all of medicine, continually advance and improve. Continuous epidural anesthesia in obstetrics is now the norm although anesthesiologists are mostly involved in a supervisory mode in delegating its administration to well trained nurse anesthetists. New anesthetics are longer lasting, requiring less frequent dosing and providing pain relief without profound muscle weakness (so called "walking epidurals"), which allow the patient to push and assist the delivery, providing the new mother with a feeling of accomplishment.

Increasingly, obstetricians are employed by hospitals and on salary. Many complain that they cannot take the time to get to know the patient as their predecessors did. I encourage them to take the time as they are missing out on much gratification, as well as missing opportunities to learn from their patients.

Communication and professionalism are now required learning in residency programs, and the practice of these skills increases patient satisfaction, fostering rapport. This should result in greater trust and fewer liability actions.

ABOUT THE AUTHOR

Dr. Eban Rock, a pseudonym for the author, was in private practice as an obstetrician and gynecologist for 34 years. As a member of the American College of Obstetrics and Gynecology, he was also a Diplomate of the American Board of Obstetrics and Gynecology. In a second career after retirement, he served as a site visitor to evaluate residency training programs applying for accreditation.

Happily retired, he is now engaged in a life-long hobby.